The *Swing!*

*Lose the Fat and Get Fit
with This Revolutionary
Kettlebell Program*

Tracy Reifkind

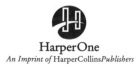

HarperOne
An Imprint of HarperCollinsPublishers

This book is written as a source of information only. The information contained in this book should by no means be considered a substitute for the advice of a qualified medical professional, who should always be consulted before beginning any new diet, exercise, or other health program.

All efforts have been made to ensure the accuracy of the information contained in this book as of the date published. The author and the publisher expressly disclaim responsibility for any adverse effects arising from the use or application of the information contained herein.

HarperOne

THE SWING! *Lose the Fat and Get Fit with This Revolutionary Kettlebell Program.* Copyright © 2012 by Tracy Reifkind. All rights reserved. Printed in the United States of America. No part of this book may be used or reproduced in any manner whatsoever without written permission except in the case of brief quotations embodied in critical articles and reviews. For information, address HarperCollins Publishers, 10 East 53rd Street, New York, NY 10022.

HarperCollins books may be purchased for educational, business, or sales promotional use. For information, please write: Special Markets Department, HarperCollins Publishers, 10 East 53rd Street, New York, NY 10022.

HarperCollins website: http://www.harpercollins.com

HarperCollins®, ▒®, and HarperOne™ are trademarks of HarperCollins Publishers.

FIRST EDITION

Designed by Terry McGrath

Photography by Victoria Yee

Library of Congress Cataloging-in-Publication Data is available upon request.

ISBN 978-0-06-210419-9

12 13 14 15 16   QGT   10 9 8 7 6 5 4 3 2 1

To my husband Mark,
the strongest man I know

Contents

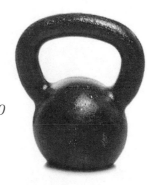

Foreword

I met Tracy Reifkind while researching remarkable stories of physical transformation for my book *The 4-Hour Body*. And what a remarkable story it was. At 250 pounds, Tracy was faced with growing health problems caused by being overweight for most of her adult life. Then, for reasons you'll learn more about, Tracy did something that few forty-one-year-olds in her position think possible—she made small, but highly effective, changes in her exercise and diet that changed *everything*. What she discovered is that one of the best-kept secrets of fat-loss, regardless of gender, is a weapon used by strong men: the kettlebell.

That wasn't the whole story. It gets much more elegant.

Even the experts underestimate the astounding effectiveness of the most fundamental kettlebell movement: *the swing*. Nothing else is necessary. Tracy's genius is in creating a program based on a dynamic progression of easy-to-follow swing movements—from beginner to master—that will transform anyone, and I don't use "transform" lightly. Together with her own inspiring story, her practical tips for shifting both your mind-set and way of eating will get you on the road to *sustainable and lasting change*. To use a technical phrase, her approach kicks serious ass.

Whether you're trying to lose the last few extra pounds or taking on a bigger challenge, just as Tracy did, *The Swing!* will make the kettlebell your new best friend and chief ally.

Give it even eight weeks and you won't recognize yourself.

Enjoy!

Tim Ferriss

author of #1 *New York Times* bestsellers
The 4-Hour Workweek and *The 4-Hour Body*

Introduction

I think about the miracle of the kettlebell each time I see my reflection in the mirror. I call it a miracle, I call it luck, and I call it finding the pot of gold. Not only did training the kettlebell swing help me lose 120 pounds at the age of forty-one after having tried just about every other type of training regimen, it made me stronger, fitter, and leaner, and it has motivated me to live up to my physical potential. I want everyone to know about it; I want everyone to fall in love with it, like I did.

First and foremost, I love the kettlebell swing because it burns more calories than any other physical activity except for uphill cross-country skiing—and who does that? I also loved the thrill of saying goodbye to hours upon hours spent every week on cardio equipment that wasn't doing a fraction of what swinging a kettlebell could help me accomplish in thirty minutes or less, just a couple days a week. The swing combines strength training and cardio fitness, and it gave me something I never had before: cardio strength endurance . . . oh, and some killer shoulders, arms, and abs! You won't get all that from a StairMaster.

In *The Swing!*, I am going to teach you how to transform your own life by swinging a kettlebell and establishing smarter eating habits. You can do this, and you don't need to wait for some professional team to come along and save you, or pay $1,000 a month for a personal trainer to help you change your body—your chance has arrived right now, in the form of this book.

I'm confident you're going to fall for the kettlebell swing just as I did. Yes, the kettlebell is the only piece of equipment you'll ever need to transform your body. And, sure, you can swing it at home—outside on your patio, in the living room or even the hallway, or out in the garage, where I started training and still train to this day. Yes, that means you will never have to step foot in a gym again (or pay for a gym membership that you never use). But the best part of the kettlebell is that it's fun. At least it is when you swing it, which I'm going to teach you to do. Here are a few more reasons why you're going to love it:

It feels natural. The swing is a primal motion that is not evoked in any other exercise program. Whether you're uncoordinated or an agile athlete, you will pick up the movement quickly. This is partially because the swing is one of the first motions our bodies are exposed to in childhood: we're rocked to sleep, lulled by the soothing motion, and we've spent hours on the playground swings as we were growing up. Yet the kettlebell swing is no lullaby or a mere thrill ride—it'll infuse you with energy and strength. No matter what your fitness background, it'll feel exhilarating.

It's no dumbbell. If you think you've tried the kettlebell because you've tried lifting weights, think again. There are plenty of static movements that you can do with a kettlebell that are similar to those done with a dumbbell. What you can't do with a dumbbell is swing it— the kettlebell handle gives it an advantage over every other form of weight-resistance exercise.

You get two workouts in one. The kettlebell swing is both aerobic and anaerobic, so you get strength and cardio in one workout. The result is an unmatched potential for cardio conditioning and fat loss. Unless you start running an hour of six-minute miles or climbing up a hill on skis, you won't find a higher caloric burn.

You will not get bored. When I started training with the swing, I thought there was no way I could stick with one movement to change my body without getting bored. So I started choreographing combinations that would keep me busy, entertained, and distracted from the repetition of a single movement. I discovered an endless possibility for combinations that build endurance and work capacity while promoting body transformation in record time.

In *The Swing!*, I'm also going to teach you how to feed yourself, because even the highest caloric burn can't out-burn overeating! To reveal the amazing tone and shape you're going to create with the swing, you've got to also strip away any extra weight you have on your body.

When people ask me how I lost all my extra weight, I often tell them I stopped doing what was making me fat. I was an extreme overeater— I was eating more than four times what I eat now, sometimes up to 5,000 calories a day. It doesn't take nearly that much to have extra fat on your body, which is why the first tenet of the Swing Diet is to lower your calories. Don't let the low-calorie initiative fool you, though—I still love to eat, so I created a diet that allows you to add volume to your plate while significantly cutting calories.

The Essential Combination

So there it is: swing a kettlebell + eat fewer calories – the essential combination for body transformation (this applies whether you want to lose 15 pounds or more than 100). You might be thinking it doesn't sound all that groundbreaking, but here's why this combination has an advantage over everything else you've ever tried: it creates real, visible results quickly—as soon as after the first four workouts.

Before I discovered the swing, I had spent decades trying various types of exercise and different diets, and *nothing* ever clicked for me. I didn't see results fast enough to create momentum or to get me permanently into the rhythm of living a healthier, fitter lifestyle. Being married to an athlete, I had witnessed plenty of people around me who had long ago picked up the rhythm and never looked back—their diet and exercise habits were so ingrained into their lives that they weren't even challenged by their weight (you know the type—those friends or family members of yours who seem to have missed the memo saying, "Weight loss is a universal struggle").

I came to the conclusion that truly healthy and fit people don't have to think about how to become healthy and fit, it's who they are—it's not a chore, a punishment, or even a choice. Forget second nature; for them, it is *first* nature. The question for me then became: how do you make something first nature?

I didn't experience an instantaneous flip of a switch when I first started swinging the kettlebell and making all of my own foods. But after just four swing sessions, I noticed something that supercharged my motivation—it wasn't just a feeling, but something I saw in a dressing room mirror: my sculpted shoulders and toned triceps, my body being transformed from chubby and soft to fit and firm. And from that point on, I never looked back. I kept swinging, I kept eating well, and I never felt like I had to sacrifice anything. I was no longer trying so hard to change my body—I had picked up the rhythm, I had found the key to creating habits that became first nature!

After so many years of trying to figure it all out, I realized it's really incredibly simple—no one wants to stick with something that doesn't produce results. I can tell you about my results from the kettlebell swing: I lost 120 pounds and have kept it off for six years; I went from a size 24 to a size 6; I used to get tired from just walking around a mall, but now I have inexhaustible energy. But I'd also like to show you what my starting point really looked like:

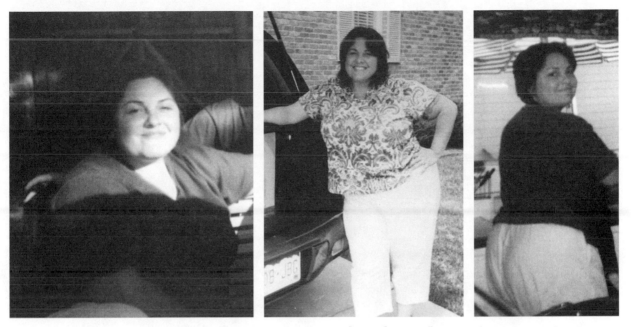

This is me before I lost 120 pounds and went from a size 24 to a size 6!

Now it's your turn to pick up the kettlebell swing and finally get the results you've always wanted. If you're tired of wasting time at the gym, sweating through step classes, logging hours on the treadmill, getting beat up in some boot camp, or jumping up and down in your living room to a useless DVD—if you're ready to finally see the results that will inspire and motivate you like never before—I invite you to try the swing!

PART ONE

Mind

The Great Discovery: Hope

"My name is Tracy Reifkind, and over the last year, I have maintained a weight loss of 120 pounds. I'm forty-three years old, 130 pounds, and 20 percent body fat, size 6." That's how my story started in 2006.

Now, several years later, I can say that not only have I maintained my weight loss but also that on the verge of turning fifty, my body is better than ever. I feel strong, sexy, and confident, and I have more energy than I did in my twenties. And it all started with one swing of a kettlebell.

The kettlebell swing changed my body in a way nothing else ever did or—I'm convinced now—ever could. I lost a lot of weight, but I had lost weight before. What I hadn't ever done was fallen in love with my body, from the way it looked to how it made me feel each day. In fact, up until I discovered the swing, I felt a complete disconnect from my body—like there was a very good chance that I had ended up in a fat body that didn't really belong to me.

I knew that inside, buried under the walls of flesh that I had put up around myself, there lurked a better version of me. I knew that inside there existed the most incredible, dynamic, and strong woman. I knew that I was a living and breathing example of unrealized potential.

And I know that's where you are now. Most likely, you don't have more than 100 pounds to lose, like I did—maybe your goal is to finally lose 20 pounds or 60, or to simply increase your strength, or to get great-looking arms—but you are filled with a voice that says, "You're not as amazing as you could be."

In *The Swing!*, I'm going to give you the program that will allow you to trade that thought in for this one: "I don't want anybody's body but my own." Jennifer Aniston? "Nope." Jessica Alba? "Nah, I like my body, thanks." That's where I am now; I wouldn't trade my body in for the world. It took me decades to be able to say that, but you're not going to have to wait that long—the path for your very own transformation exists right here in this book.

It's All in the Rhythm

It should come as no surprise that to get on the path to body transformation, you have to incorporate exercise and establish smarter eating habits. It sounds so simple, and yet just about everyone seems to be frustrated with weight or a lack of bodily control. I tried countless times to lose weight, but I could never stick with anything—I felt like I was always fighting the changes I had to make; they never felt natural.

That all changed when I discovered the kettlebell swing and learned how to feed myself nourishing, fulfilling, and delicious foods. When I discovered this combination, I realized that when the formula is right, the solution comes easily. And the formula isn't even a complicated one—it involves methods that will feel very familiar, even natural, to you.

The motion of the swing itself draws on a very soothing, almost meditative flow that feels comfortable, instead of restrictive or forced. The rhythm of the exercise—the back and forth of the weight, like a pendulum—puts you in touch with your body, and it reminds you that your muscles were made to move. I know it may seem hard to believe that I'm talking about exercise, but just wait until you try it!

Not only does the motion of the kettlebell swing feel right, it also provides the most intense calorie burn without requiring a significant time investment. There's a complicated explanation (see page 61) for the swing's incomparable efficiency, but the simplest way to explain it is to say that it's like getting a two-for-one deal—even though you're doing just one exercise, you're actually getting the benefits and caloric burn of two types of exercise: strength training and cardiovascular conditioning.

Part of the beauty of creating an aerobic and anaerobic workout at the same time is that you get the benefits of both. Your kettlebell swings will help you build strength and create muscle tone, improve muscle endurance and lung capacity, and build power and explosiveness for other sports and activities. And without a doubt, they will accelerate fat burn, helping you reveal visible results in as little as four swing sessions. I still remember the first time I saw my new body taking shape—it was an unforgettable turning point for me.

The Girl in the Mirror

I had been doing the kettlebell swing for only a few weeks when I first noticed results. I was in a department store dressing room where I was trying on a pair of jeans, and I saw something in the mirror that stopped me in my tracks. The motion of pulling up a pair of smaller-sized jeans revealed a shoulder and triceps muscle tone that didn't seem familiar on my body; it had to belong to an athlete or at the very least a fit woman. I had been 250 pounds for the last ten years of my life—this couldn't possibly be my body, but it was. To see this shape on my own body was a life-changing vision—my true body was breaking through.

Up until that point in my life, I had felt my body wasn't my own. Even as a kid, I was chubby—I didn't know what it felt like to do a cartwheel or to hang from the monkey bars, or to enjoy any other popular childhood activities. In my twenties, I tried just about everything to change my body: weight lifting, different types of cardio, diet foods, diet pills . . . you name it.

I got especially into bodybuilding during the '80s and even became a regular at Gold's Gym, performing my shoulder raises, bicep curls, and chest presses like a mad woman. Still, I never saw so much as a toned arm. (I would say that all my hours at that gym were wasted, but

The Truth About Gyms

Most exercise machines at the gym will not help you lose weight. Think about it—how many overweight people do you see at the average gym? Not many. Most of the people you see there have already lost weight and are working out to maintain their fitness. Those who have more than 10 pounds to lose won't stick around long because they just will not see the results they're hoping for. Here's why: with gym machines, you don't burn enough calories to create significant change in your weight, let alone to reveal muscle or tone. If the average person jogs on the treadmill for thirty minutes, he will have burned about 130 calories; two bites of a Snickers candy bar, and you're right back to where you started.

When you learn the kettlebell swing, you're going to more than double that caloric burn, working your way up to torching nearly 300 calories in just twenty minutes. Keep in mind that even with a burn like that, the importance of diet doesn't disappear—it's an essential companion to exercise, always and forever.

that wouldn't be true—I met the love of my life there!) As I gained and lost weight over the years, my body only got smaller or bigger, never shapelier.

In my thirties, I only seemed to get bigger, gaining weight steadily through the decade. By forty-one, my body was tired and beat up, my insides and internal organs were swimming in fatty tissue, my face was bloated and saggy, my energy dragging each day.

I became convinced that I was always going to have a problem with my weight. I chalked it up to genetics—a fit, healthy body just wasn't in my genes. Other women could create a bikini body, gorgeous strong arms, or a flat tummy, but not me. So you can imagine how startling it was to see beautiful shape developing in my body.

When I saw myself in the mirror, I knew right then and there that I had the kettlebell swings to thank because nothing else I had ever tried had produced this effect. The swing had begun to transform my body, and the results were so undeniable and impressive, I was more motivated than ever to keep going.

Hungry for More . . . Results

When I first started training with the swing, it hadn't been implemented as the core activity in any exercise program. Athletes and military crews were using it as part of a cross-training program, but no one was using it as a stand-alone exercise. It seemed strange to me that the most perfect exercise was only being used as a small part of a larger session rather than being treated as the star it was.

After time, I discovered that the one movement of the swing could be designed into many different combinations using just your two hands. One movement + one bell = endless variety. I set out to choreograph combinations that would keep me busy, entertained, and distracted from the repetition of only one movement, all the while building endurance and work capacity, and promoting an unmatched potential for cardio conditioning and fat loss. The result: an unbeatable workout that promotes body transformation in record time.

Once I created my own swing progressions for my workouts, there was no stopping me. My personal results were so incredible that I knew I had to teach others, which meant becoming a certified kettlebell trainer. I obtained my RKC (Russian Kettlebell Certification) and started actively blogging my workout routines and creating video demonstrations of my workout methods. Quite a few people started following my routines rep for rep, just doing the workouts as I had written them out online. I was having so much fun doing my own swing routines that I started teaching them in person, and the feedback was incredible, which eventually led to creating DVDs of the workouts. I couldn't believe my personal transformation had led to such amazing opportunities—and I'm still pinching myself.

I also started to create customized nutrition plans for my clients because no matter how many swings you do, you simply cannot out-train your food intake. If you're not fueling your body with the right foods or, if your goal is weight loss, if you're not eating fewer calories, you cannot create the body you want. There's no way around this fact, but there is a way to eat that will ensure the momentum you create with your swings will continue right on into the kitchen.

The Uncommon Common-Sense Diet

The Swing Diet is the essential companion to your kettlebell swings. I've created it to give your body the support it needs to shed fat and develop muscle tone as you complete your workouts. To ensure the diet is fully ingrained into your life, I'm going to teach you skills that will help you get into the rhythm of preparing your own foods, helping you to take true ownership of your transformation.

The eating plan in this book is all about smart and simple diet strategies; it's not complicated or expensive, and it doesn't require you to buy any specialized supplements. I like to think of it as the Uncommon Common Sense Diet because it's based on what we all know but choose to forget.

When I started designing the diet for myself, I knew three things for sure: 1) I had to make and prepare all of my own foods—no more eating out; 2) I needed to feel completely satisfied, because I still had the mind-set of an overeater; and 3) I needed flavor! No flavorless or bland foods allowed. Essentially, I needed to be able to eat a lot of food that tasted good and could be made at home. These may seem like obvious requirements, but if you've ever tried "diet" foods you know that plentiful and tasty are not commonly used descriptions. Staying on a diet you don't like won't work, which is why in Part Three I will teach you how to eat to change your body by filling your plate with plenty of food and flavor.

There are millions of very frustrated people out there who spend hours working out but don't change their diet and then wonder why their weight doesn't budge—don't be one of them. Unless you change what you're eating, you will not change your body. For me, acknowledging the significance of diet marked one of the biggest turning points in my body transformation.

It's Not a Weight Issue

Like most people, I used to think what I had most of my life was a weight issue, but I realized finally that when it really came down to it, what I had was a food—or eating—issue. It's a cause-and-effect relationship—my weight was a problem, but what was creating the excess weight was all the food I was eating that my body did not need. It's safe to say I was eating too many calories.

Here were a couple of my favorite lunches: three McDonald's cheeseburgers, six chocolate chip cookies, and a large soda = 2,170 calories; or six Jack in the Box tacos, an order of curly fries, and a large root beer = 2,137 calories. The fast-food joints were about fifteen minutes from my home, and all that food was gone before my front tires hit my driveway. Sometimes I even had time to stop at the gas station for a couple of packs of Hostess Donuts (an additional 400 calories per package). It's no mystery why I was fat.

It's also not shocking that the general population is getting fatter and fatter—the average daily consumption is nearly 4,000 calories, when it should be less than 2,000 for most women. If you are overweight, you are consuming more calories than you need to fuel your body properly for its daily functions. It's science, but it's not rocket science.

It's time to stop filling your body with food*stuff*—processed foods, snacks, junk foods—and to discover what it feels like to eat whole-food-based meals that give energy and life rather than take it away. I used to be so disconnected from the purpose and the pleasure of real food that I consumed thousands upon thousands of empty calories each day for years. But why was I compelled to eat so much? Because I could, just as we all can. It felt like the ultimate luxury to eat whatever I wanted, and I couldn't stop myself from taking advantage of the abundance and availability of food.

The truth is, it's not a luxury when you take an honest look at the effects overeating has on your body. All that extra food you're "treating" yourself with equals extra weight, and that takes a serious toll on your body.

Unless you live under a rock, you know that being overweight has been linked to a number of diseases. What you may not know is that the extra weight also does a number on your knee joints, with each pound equaling about four pounds of pressure on your knees. That means when I was 250, I made my body work so much harder than it had to—adding close to 500 pounds of extra work to every move I made. Doesn't sound so luxurious now, does it?

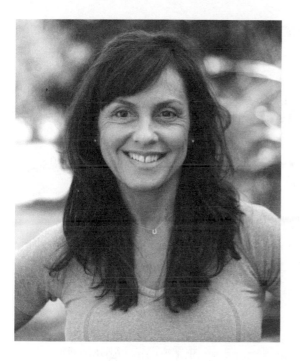

Real luxury comes in the form of fueling your body with rich, delicious foods that also happen to be healthful. Fresh, whole foods fuel your cells and fill your body with energizing oxygen. Creating a direct connection with these types of foods—preparing them and cooking them for yourself—is one of the vital keys to weight loss. It doesn't have to be difficult either; in Part Three of this book, I'll teach you smart strategies that will help you quickly get into the rhythm of making your own meals. Eating well can be a deeply satisfying and rewarding experience, but it doesn't have to become a full-time job.

Weight Time

Rarely do I have a client come to me who can say exactly what his or her weight is—and this is not by accident. When I was overweight, I didn't even own a scale or a full-length mirror. Research shows that there's a significant difference between measured and self-reported weight, especially among overweight individuals. It's time to put denial to rest and step on the scale. This will be one of the most important steps in establishing your starting point (for specifics on tracking your weight loss, see page 43), but be sure not to confuse your weight with your identity. Your weight is a reflection of the amount of calories you eat, period. In fact, as you begin, I want you to evaluate and remind yourself of your personal strengths that have nothing to do with weight. Getting back in touch with these strengths will boost your confidence and will give you a great foundation on which to build.

The Perfect Plan for Real Life

Sometimes it seems the workouts and diets featured in books and magazines were created by people who never tried to lose weight; I am not one of those people. I've tried it all, which is why I have such confidence in the program I've designed for you. After years of trying and failing to change my body, I used the workouts and eating plans featured in this book to lose 120 pounds and to keep it off.

The swing worked for me because it's the most authentic and direct path to transformation—when you swing the kettlebell and fuel your body with simple, whole foods, it will feel like a revelation, like you've finally discovered the most natural and true way to create the body you've always wanted.

With a promise like that, I'm sure you're eager to jump right to the workouts and the diet, but I encourage you to read the rest of Part One first. My own personal evolution to the point where it finally clicked for me took twenty years—from that process, I produced gems of insight that I share with my personal clients, and now I'm going to share them with you.

2 Reconnecting with Your Body

Being a formerly fat person, I know what it feels like to see your body as an other; some part of you from which you've disconnected. When you are disconnected from your body, your thoughts and perceptions of your body don't match reality. If you've ever had a moment when you looked in a mirror and thought, "How is that possibly what my body looks like?" you know what I'm talking about.

Weight gain—as little as 10 pounds—happens when you stop paying attention and start disconnecting from your physical body. It can start innocently, say, over the holidays or on a cruise, when you've given yourself a break to stop thinking about what you're eating or how little you're exercising. (Don't even get me started on how ridiculous this thinking is to begin with—we should be taking a break from overeating, not the other way around!)

Next thing you know, you've added 10 pounds. And then, since you gained that 10 pounds, why not just let yourself go a bit more? Tack on another 15. This weight may take many years to accumulate, but let me tell you, the timing doesn't work in your favor. Pretty soon, you're over forty and your metabolism's slowed down, your muscle mass is dwindling, and you're staring at a big number that you want to cut off your weight. That's certainly where I ended up.

What happens when you get to that point is you begin to exist in the space outside of your body—the space where you can deny the physical and mental damage you are causing yourself and instead swim in the false and temporary pleasure of overeating. This space isn't all ice cream and candy bars, though—in fact, it's filled with thoughts and feelings of guilt and shame, feelings so powerful that they take over, and you become your thoughts, emotions, and doubts. When you exist so much in this intangible kind of headspace, reconnecting with your body can feel really uncomfortable, even a bit painful.

When I say painful, I don't mean just the physical pain of muscle soreness (although there will be some of that too), but the disappointment and frustration that comes with acknowledging the undeniable fact that you have let yourself get out of shape. Exercising brings you back into your body, which, if you are overweight, is not a comfortable place to find yourself.

The best way to deal with this transition is to stop thinking and start doing—you are going to be amazed at how quickly your pain turns into power. There's no time like right now to start to bridge the gap between your mind and body, between your actions and your expectations. And here's why the kettlebell swing is the absolute best exercise to lead this charge: there's no waiting around for the effects; you will feel your body come to life the moment you start swinging.

When you begin with the swing, you will become reacquainted with your body instantaneously. The motion itself engages just about every muscle on your body, from your triceps to your inner thighs to the many muscle fibers that make up your core. This doesn't even count the cardiovascular challenge that will kick in within seconds and spike your oxygen intake, invigorating your cells and muscle tissues and improving blood circulation.

The instant impact of the kettlebell swing is revitalizing, but when you keep swinging, the rewards get even greater. The first gift is a renewed connection to your body, and soon to follow is the introduction to your *new body*. You will begin to see signs of your new body in as little as four twenty- to thirty-minute workouts—that means real, visible changes that will start to show up in the mirror in just a couple of hours. There is no other type of exercise that can make this promise—not running, weight lifting, hiking, aerobics, or anything else.

Walk, Don't Run

If you aren't ready to jump onto the fast track to results with the swing workouts, you can begin with walking. Before I started swinging the kettlebell, I walked not because I thought it would provoke the weight loss I wanted but because it allowed me to get back in touch with my body. Walking helps you remember what it feels like just to put your body to work—it's like a mediator who will restart the conversation between your mind and body.

Walking is also the best gauge for a basic level of fitness for a person of any weight or age, and it's a much smarter beginning activity than running. I've seen many people try running for weight loss, and two things usually happen: 1) they get injured, and 2) they don't lose any weight. It takes a lot of training and cardiovascular fitness to get to the point where running is beneficial for you. Bottom line, you get in shape to run, you don't run to get in shape.

Walking works. It doesn't matter how slow you have to go—you can take the first step toward change right now. You may not be on the fast track yet, but you are on the track and just getting there can be the toughest part of all.

The Body and Its Capacity for Forgiveness

When you start swinging the kettlebell and reconnecting with your body, you might experience your body holding a grudge—getting sore, making life feel difficult for you—but I have good news: no matter what shape you're in now, your body is ready to forgive you and reward you for the changes you are about to make to your daily habits. Despite all the workouts you've missed, the crap you've eaten, and the pounds you've added, it is never too late to create the body you've always dreamed of. My story proves this.

I tried to lose weight countless times over the years—and I spent plenty of years bouncing back and forth between weights. I tried Jenny Craig and lost 20 pounds, and then regained them and about 20 more. I took tae kwon do with my son and lost weight, and then gained again.

This type of repeated weight gain and weight loss is often referred to as yo-yo dieting, but it's not a game. In fact, it's thought to contribute to heart problems and high cholesterol, and it has shown to actually slow metabolism, which makes it especially difficult to maintain any weight loss.

Yet the most significant impact of yo-yo dieting is the emotional roller coaster it creates. Gaining weight is depressing; losing weight is invigorating—and no one is happy when they are constantly bouncing back and forth between these extreme emotions. It creates a kind of double existence, and it keeps you from ever feeling completely comfortable or happy.

Eventually you give up, talking yourself into accepting the alternating weight loss and gain as a fact of life. Still, over time, small weight gain becomes bigger gain, which makes it more likely you'll get stuck at the higher number on the scale, instead of the lower. That's what happened to me—I started putting on 20 pounds a year until I had gone from a size 14 to a size 24 in just five years. By forty-one, I was 250 pounds, and it seemed that's where I was going to stay. If I had done nothing, I would have kept gaining—350 pounds was right around the corner.

By some miracle, no serious obesity-related health issues caught up with me. I was certainly pre-diabetic, but I never knew for sure though how bad off I was health-wise because I avoided going to the doctor for years. I was in such denial, I couldn't bear to face the truth.

I did start snoring very loudly, which was extremely embarrassing, and I knew it was because of my weight. I also took a devastating fall after a misplaced step on a rock. The intense force of my weight as it smashed my knees into the ground overwhelmed me, and I started sobbing. The pain was severe, but I also remember the shock and horror of feeling the huge load of my body hit the ground.

Remarkably, my body recovered—from that fall and from all the years of being ignored and neglected, treated mostly just as a receptacle for useless, empty calories. My swing workouts and new eating habits picked me up off the ground and transformed me into a person unrecognizable from the one I was before. Instead of dragging though each day, I started feeling excited to be in my body; I felt energized and

What's Your Wake-Up Call?

You don't have to be nearly as heavy as I was to experience something that triggers you to want to change your habits. Research shows most people finally change their health habits because of something medical—often either a doctor telling them to lose weight or a family member having a heart attack. The next most common triggering events have been reported as "reaching an all-time high in weight" or "seeing a picture or reflection." I think the last one is certainly something just about everyone can relate to! So you have a choice: you can either wait for one of these messages to come along, or you can accept the chance I'm giving you in The Swing! *to create momentum and results in just a few short weeks. You've got nothing to lose but weight.*

enthusiastic about life. Instead of feeling completely disconnected from the me I saw in the mirror, I started falling in love with my body, and it started loving me back, giving me the invaluable gift of health.

In the end, what I discovered is that our bodies are not indestructible, but they are repairable and recoverable. This is true regardless of your current shape. Whether you're a few years out of college, post-baby, entering menopause, fighting middle-aged weight gain, facing a weight loss of more than 100 pounds, or you've simply grown tired of that stubborn 20 pounds, the swing will propel you toward your desired body transformation. The first step for everyone is the same—to swing the kettlebell, thereby starting the conversation with your body. Maybe say a thank-you to your body for enduring your past indulgences, and then make a commitment moving forward to reward it with the gift of good health.

3 *Get Over It!*

I always knew I could lose weight, I just didn't know when.
As my thirties flew by and I turned forty, I started to wonder if "when" was ever going to arrive. Maybe I was just
going to be fat for the rest of my life. I didn't know anyone
who had lost a tremendous amount of weight, kept it off,
and looked better than ever, regardless of his or her age.
I began to believe permanent weight loss wasn't possible.

That all changed when I discovered the kettlebell. My entire life—my
notions of what was possible with my body and my self-confidence, my
understanding of the ceiling of my capabilities, my definition of life
change—all of it was rewritten completely when I picked up a kettlebell
and started doing the kettlebell swing. I didn't just lose weight, but I
also discovered my true self along the way.

Everyone has a definition of his or her true self—it's usually the best
version of ourselves; the one we wish will show up on the most
important days of our lives. What the kettlebell swing helped me
realize is that the best you doesn't have to be a guest star; you can be
who you've always wanted to be every day—there's no reason to keep
all that greatness locked up inside!

• •

The Inside Truth

Ever since I was a little kid, I've envied athletes. I've always admired their sense of purpose and the control they have over their bodies. When I would envision my dream body, I would see myself fit, athletic, and shapely; I never wanted to be just skinny. I also saw in athletes a reflection of my true self—the self that was driven, capable, and strong, filled with a competitive spirit that could persevere through challenges and always stay the course.

It took me years to bring the athlete inside of me to life, but once I did, the reality matched my dreams (and even exceeded them). Identifying and knowing the characteristics of your true self can be an important step in helping the real you break through. Can you identify the qualities of your best potential self? Start to construct the physical and mental profile of who you want to be; the more solid this vision becomes, the more likely you are to make it manifest.

• •

Fortunately, you're the one who holds the key to unlocking your own lasting transformation. To make it happen, you've first got to get out of the pit of unrealized potential—the slick and oily collection of all the excuses you've used to keep yourself from making progress until now. The pit is covered in thoughts like this:

I'm too old.

I'm too fat.

I have a thyroid problem.

I have a slow metabolism.

I've had children (it ruined my body).

I have children (they consume my life).

I work full time.

I'm so tired.

It's Monday.

It's Friday.

I have to go shopping.

I know you've convinced yourself that it's okay to stay trapped in excuses like these. You've probably also had people in your life validate them, but I've got news for you: I'm not one of those people. The truth is, you are limiting yourself in unimaginable ways if you continue to settle for a life filled with excuses. Breaking free from all these unproductive, wasteful, fallback positions all starts with one statement: I am in control.

The Power of Control

When you claim control of your life and the daily choices you make, you silence excuses and blame, and you ensure that you'll never play victim to anything ever again. If you've ever pointed a finger at something or someone else and blamed him, her, or it for the current state of your body, then you have given up control. Worse, you happen to be in the comfortable company of many.

Real vs. Fake

When I was heavy, I used to make an effort to control perceptions of myself. I wasn't about to let people perceive me as fat and foolish, so I practically bragged about taking responsibility for my weight. At the full-service salon where I worked, I was the first one to go get fast food for myself and everyone else, and I openly helped myself to the Saturday morning tray of donuts. I would boast about eating the most fattening ice creams, the most fattening foods, and how if I was going to be fat, I might as well thoroughly enjoy all the junk foods I could get my hands on. In reality, I felt like a bottomless pit; my control was nonexistent, and the act was pointless because it only perpetuated my own weight gain. It was only when I was finally honest with myself that I was ready to take authentic control of my life—I wasn't proud of being fat, so why was I pretending to be?

Take a personal inventory of the efforts you make to seem like something you're not. Plenty of people, especially women, will take on this attitude of having fat pride—but I know it's a lie. Being overweight not only places limits on your life, it puts your health on the line, which is nothing to brag about. Real control is about taking ownership of your health and body, and making sure your actions are those that will bring to life your true desires.

The act of blaming something other than ourselves for what goes wrong is casually encouraged in our culture, so much so that we often don't even bother to consider another explanation for our predicament. Even most of the weight-loss books out there will play into your desire to find a scapegoat . . . *it's carbs; it's fat; you're not doing enough cardio; you're not eating enough whole grains; you're eating the wrong foods for your body type.* No one seems to want to say the one true thing, which is that it's your fault. You are responsible for the shape you're in. You are eating more calories than your body needs, and your body is storing them as fat. It wasn't until I accepted this fact that I was able to create a profound change in my life.

If there is one influence that will keep you from losing that first pound, it is continuing to blame your weight on anyone or anything other than yourself. Then, of course, for every excuse out there, there is a person who has beaten it. Ultimately, your body will not change until you change your habits and behavior. I've created a few rules that will help you set these changes in motion.

Regaining Control with Rules

You put yourself in control of your health by taking two important steps: First, you recognize that you have the power to choose what you put in your mouth. Second, acknowledge that you have the ability to determine how much you exercise and to devise a program to attain your goals. This is a no-brainer, but it brings us back to the golden rule of change, which is that to create change, you must first accept control.

Beyond that, there are a few other solid rules that I discovered on the path to body transformation. These are rooted in science and are as inevitable as sunrise each day. As my husband, Mark, likes to say, "I don't make the rules; I just know 'em." I love this phrase because it reminds me that there are some undeniable truths when it comes to how your body works—knowing these will take a lot of guesswork out of the equation and will boost confidence in your control. I'll go into these in more detail in later chapters, but here are the most basic rules about body transformation:

- **Forget everything else you've been told; it's all about calories.** Make no mistake; it's pure science. If you eat fewer calories than you burn on any given day, you will lose weight.

- **Guessing doesn't cut it.** You must educate yourself by tracking your calories, not because you're monitoring restriction, but because you're tracking progress. Everyone underestimates the amount of food he or she eats each day. In fact, studies have shown that people can underestimate their calorie consumption up to 42 percent—that's like eating 3,000 calories but thinking you've eaten a little over 1,700 calories. You will never lose weight unless you have a clear picture of what you're eating.

- **The kettlebell swing is the most effective method for rapid weight loss.** A study conducted by the American Council on Exercise revealed that a kettlebell workout burns up to 20.2 calories per minute. To achieve this kind of caloric burn in any other activity, you would have to be an extreme athlete. It's the equivalent of running a six-minute mile, which is almost impossible for the average adult, but everyone can swing a kettlebell!

These are indisputable rules—there's no gray area or room for discussion. When you accept these rules, you will empower yourself with basic body truths. Use them as general guidelines and come back to them often, especially if you ever feel your commitment to change grow shaky. The rules won't change, which means they'll never fail to keep you—or get you back—on track.

How Small, Smart Changes Can Lead to Big Results

Let's say you've set your excuses aside and kicked the blame game to the curb. What's the next step? Personally, I wasn't planning for perfection from the get-go, but instead for what was possible for me to achieve, one step at a time. I lost the first 50 pounds by changing my diet. I knew that at some point I would have to add weight-resistance training, but I needed to focus on one change at a time. I wasn't aiming to accomplish amazing results quickly, but I soon realized that it was possible.

I started slowly with the kettlebell swing, doing just five to ten minutes twice a week, but the confidence I gained from just being able to do that much helped build my motivation. With motivation came commitment to my workouts, which led to continued results. Each action or change I made built upon the one that had come before it—it was a chain reaction that, once set in motion, couldn't be stopped. And it continues today as I complete my kettlebell workouts and prep and cook my meals each week—it's all part of who I am now.

To set yourself on the same track, there are very basic steps to follow: make changes, aim for results, and build on the motivation from meeting your goals. When in doubt about your diet, always return to calories and your honest account of what foods you're putting in your body—this is the most reliable way to monitor your progress. And with exercise, just follow this simple rule my husband taught me: swing the kettlebell until you break a sweat and then stop. (It's a trick of course; because once you break a sweat all you'll want to do is keep going.)

When it comes to changing our habits, we all feel as if we have mighty demons to face and huge obstacles to overcome in order to make commitments stick, but let's not waste more time looking for excuses. You deserve to be great, and it's time for you to accept that you can be. Embrace control by taking personal responsibility for the choices you make and by filtering those choices through the rules of body transformation. Do this and I guarantee you will create the changes you want to see in your body and your life.

The Right Mind-Set

A big mistake many people make is that when they start a diet and exercise program, they fail to see it as a permanent lifestyle change. That was a mistake I made for years—all the diet and exercise methods I tried were just temporary fixes that never really became a part of my regular life. They came and went like passing trends tend to do, and my weight responded in kind, fluctuating and then flatlining at fat.

Then I started paying more attention to my husband's habits (I had made subconscious observations over the years, but they had never crossed over into my own habits). He was and still is the perpetual athlete, methodical about his diet and training regimens without fail. His body responded, too, by getting stronger and leaner, and barely ever varying in weight over the twenty-plus years I've known him. I couldn't even fathom having such power over my body.

What I realized is that he had a wildly different mind-set from my own—I had the average mind-set, and he had the athlete's mind-set. If the average mind-set operates from the kind of inconsistency that creates yo-yo dieting, the athlete's mind-set thrives on the opposite: consistency. It's not about exercising or eating well every once in a while, but about making those practices part of your everyday life. Athletes know this instinctively, but for most people it doesn't come naturally. The incredible lesson I learned is that you don't have to be an athlete to think like one—in fact, anyone and everyone can take cues from an athlete's way of thinking to help create and keep the body you've always wanted.

It all comes down to getting into the Readiness Zone.

The Readiness Zone

Athletes connect everything they do to the body—they have an image and an idea of the shape they'd like to be in, and they eat and exercise accordingly to bring this image to life. Their regimens are designed to maximize performance and to make sure they're always within a certain zone of fitness, what I like to call the Readiness Zone. When they're in this zone, they're physically strong and prepared, always ready to train and within reach of their top form. They've developed habits that keep them in this zone, but it's not about the specifics of their habits as much as it is about the consistency of them. For them, there's no turning off or letting go.

For most other people, it's a constant back-and-forth between letting go and then reining back in, which means following a pattern that looks a lot like this:

▶ Eat whatever you want, exercise as little as possible, feel dissatisfied with your body, and resolve to do something about it someday.

▶ Someday comes—your clothes get too tight, you have a wedding to go to, you want to comfortably wear a bathing suit, or you've found that dream pair of jeans you're just dying to fit into.

▶ You throw yourself into some sort of rapid weight-loss plan, which usually involves something drastic or unhealthful, but you lose weight and feel great.

▶ You attend the event, you fit into the jeans, and you are sexy and confident. You think, "I am never going to gain weight again."

▶ You stop following XYZ plan because it was too restrictive and unrealistic—it just didn't fit into your life—and the pounds sneak back on.

▶ Repeat.

When you follow this type of pattern, you spend most of the time existing outside of the Readiness Zone—you are almost always tens of pounds away from being ready or prepared for whatever comes your way. Instead of feeling confident and excited for an event or the beach or even a shopping trip with your friends, there's a sense of dread and embarrassment, or a memory of how much work it's going to take to get back into the zone again. When you live your life in this space, spontaneity dies and limits live large.

There were plenty of times when my weight held me back, mentally and physically. Just being on my feet with all that extra body weight made activities like walking around an amusement park or even the mall painful. That doesn't even count the "pain" of actually shopping—trying on clothing in front of a mirror never failed to feel like torture. I couldn't wear heels; the pressure of my own body weight made them too painful to bear.

Then, there were the places I wouldn't even go because of my body—forget the beach; I didn't own a pair of shorts or a bathing suit. Once, when someone gave Mark and me a trip to Hawaii, I had to go—and I was miserable the entire time! On a free trip to Hawaii, I couldn't even enjoy myself because I was so embarrassed by how I looked. I also used to try to avoid people when I was at my heaviest—I'd stay away from the house when I knew old friends would visit, or I'd slip down a different aisle at the grocery store if I saw someone I knew. When I think about it now, I can't believe I placed such limits and restrictions on my life, or that I lived with so much shame.

Consider the limits you've placed on your own life by not being in the body you want, one that's not as fit, strong, or lean as you'd like it to be. You may not even be aware of some of the simplest things that you are missing out on or the negativity you perpetuate as a result of your weight. Are there events or gatherings you've skipped out on because you don't want people to see the weight you've gained? Have you opted not to get out on the dance floor because you can't stand the thought of people staring at your body? Have you rushed to get out of a picture so you wouldn't have to see your arms, thighs, or belly immortalized in an image? Individually, these may seem like small sacrifices, but joined together, they create a powerful anti-life force—they're pulling you out of and away from your fullest potential.

Now imagine yourself instead always ready and up for anything. See yourself perpetually in the Readiness Zone. Imagine feeling confident and excited each day, ready to take on and accept any opportunity that comes your way. What doors do you want your capable and strong body to open for you? See yourself going on a hike with your friends or taking a challenging walk without telling others to go on without you. Or envision yourself trying something exciting while on vacation, like surfing or zip-lining, or training for a 5k because you want to run one with your kids. Imagine your life free of the pattern of self-defeat created by yo-yo dieting.

That's where I am now: forever in the zone and ready to take on any adventure, the spectacular and the small. I have a renewed joy for life and an enthusiasm for being an active participant in each day. I love seeing friends, including people I haven't seen in years; I go out dancing—in heels; I try on clothes in department stores, and I get compliments on how fit I look. I have grown to love yoga and have even gotten good at it, which is something I could never do when I was heavy.

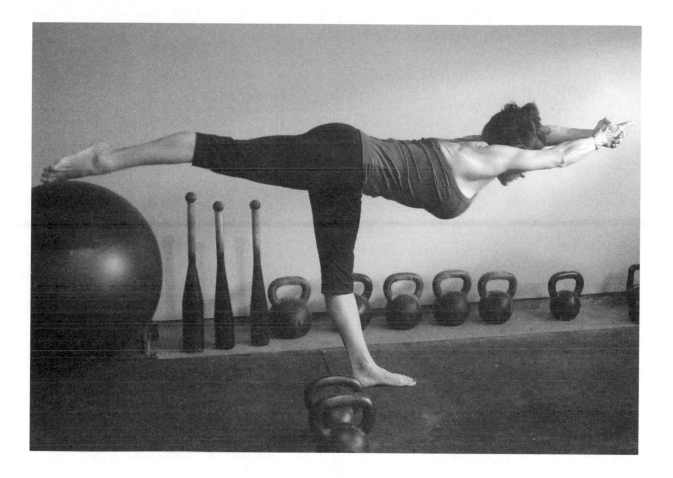

I can lead kettlebell swing classes and out-swing people half my age and even former Marines. My body is now the reason I can do what I want, not the reason I can't—and I want it to be this way for you too.

Not only is this life possible, it's easily attainable when you make the kettlebell swing and eating right part of how you live your life. Your first step in creating your own Readiness Zone is to decide to make the choices every day that support being your best at all times. At the core of how athletes live their life is the simple-sounding mantra: be consistent. I want you to adapt and imprint this phrase into your brain like a permanent tattoo. The moment you start drifting from consistency is the moment you start slipping from the Readiness Zone—tether yourself to your new habits until they become part of who you are. Be routine with your workouts and follow the eating plan daily, and you simply will not fail.

Creating Consistency

A woman once asked me how often I trained for yoga. When I told her that I had established a daily practice, she responded with amazement and was baffled by the thought of the "discipline" (her word) required to maintain that kind of commitment. So I asked her how many days she went to work. She replied: "Every day—Monday through Friday!" When I asked her if it took discipline to do that, she said that it didn't feel like discipline, it's just what she does; it's her job, and she likes her job. Exactly. Making my own foods, swinging a kettlebell, going to yoga is what I do; it's part of who I am. These are what make me feel fully alive every day.

Here are some tips on how to get onto the train of consistency—and stay there:

- **Accept the luxury of no choice.** Well, you do have a choice—you can opt to get fatter, weaker, and sicker. Let me be the first to tell you that, especially as you get older, those are your choices—you can either pursue the high road to health, or you can decline into a constant, worsening battle against your own body. This is why I like to consider it a no-choice scenario.

- **Eat the same foods at least four days out of seven.** I eat five days of the same basic meals, and then day six is my high-calorie day and day seven is my lower-calorie day. When you eat the same basic meals every day, you remove the stress that comes with choosing what foods to eat. Plus, you're able to keep more accurate calorie counts, and you become fast and efficient at preparing the same basic foods. Even if you fall off track, you won't fall far because you already have a plan for the next day.

- **Be selfish.** Have you ever been on an airplane and paid attention to the flight attendants when they are giving the safety instructions? They say something like, "If you are with a small child and the oxygen mask is released, secure your own oxygen mask first, and then give one to the child." To me, that means you'll be of no help to anyone if you die. When I was ready to change my life, I applied this strategy to my health habits. I scheduled fitness appointments with myself like they were doctor's appointments with outrageous cancellation fees.

It works—try it. Mark your calendar with the days and times of your workouts and walks, and also note when you're going to go shopping for foods and when you're going to cook them. Then, stick to this rule: nothing comes before me. Make it a priority at all costs. Wake up an hour earlier (I find this to be the easier option) or go to bed an hour later. Get rid of the riffraff in your life that doesn't support these changes.

The reality is that you have to put your health and fitness first. Establish the habits, and the body will follow, leading you right into the Readiness Zone, where limits don't exist. A nutritiously fed body that swings a kettlebell at least forty minutes a week will be one that achieves, at the very minimum, a healthy body weight. Then of course there's the swagger, the sexiness, the confidence and capability, and the complete and profound satisfaction with your body (the one you want more than anyone else's) that will come along too.

5 *The Entry Point*

I'm often asked what "it" was for me, the moment that I decided to lose the weight after so many years of going back and forth between trying and giving up. It was a sort of perfect storm of events that finally pushed me into change. My body spoke up first, then my mind, followed by a fateful triggering of my competitive side. The specifics of my evolution were unique, but the process left me with invaluable insight into the makeup of a transformation. In this chapter, I'm going give you the steps to create your very own breakthrough, but first I'm going to share a little about my own story.

A Brewing Fear

When you're more than 100 pounds overweight, your body can only go on functioning in a normal way for so long. After I had been 250 pounds for nearly ten years, I began to sense that it was about to catch up with me—and I was right. I started having digestive issues (I won't go into details, but I will tell you it wasn't pretty). I knew my body was finally speaking up in a way that I couldn't ignore. Each day for months, I felt I was dodging a bullet, but I was too scared and embarrassed to go to the doctor, so I began to self-diagnose and watch medical shows for clues.

Watching these shows only worsened my fears—I saw a story about an obese woman who died from a blood clot due to an enlarged heart. I already knew heart disease was the number-one killer of women. I was convinced my heart was swimming in fat, and I was scared that I couldn't undo the damage I had caused to my body; I was terrified I was walking the same path as the woman on TV. I knew the time had come when I had no choice but to lose weight, but my past attempts had led me to failure and left me in my current state. I was searching for the way into an overhaul of my life—and that's when the contest came along.

An Unexpected Opportunity

In the early days of January 2005, six of my co-workers decided to take on a weight-loss challenge. They were going to wager $100 per person, and whoever lost the biggest percentage of body weight would be the winner and take home the pot of collected money. I heard the conversation, but I wasn't asked to join in. I'm sure they assumed I wasn't interested in losing weight since I constantly bragged about eating whatever I wanted.

What they didn't know was that I was primed and searching for a jump-start to change and that I was a true competitor at heart. (I was a diehard *Survivor* fan and wanted so badly to compete on that show, but my extreme body weight would have made it impossible.) I jumped up from my seat and asked my co-workers to include me—they were shocked but more than happy to take my money and fatten the pot. I'm certain no one expected me to win—except me. I knew without a doubt I was going to win. I knew that I was a fireball fueled by decades of frustration with my weight—and that I was about to direct all that focus into changing my body. It was like someone had reached into the competitive switch in my brain and flipped it on—and it hasn't gone off since.

Three months later and $700 richer (I won the bet), I was a completely changed woman. I was making and preparing all my own foods, walking every day, and enjoying a wonderful, new, healthier life—and I knew I was only at the tip of the iceberg. I had lost 50 pounds already. It all started when I made the initial commitment to the weight-loss challenge, but there were critical, tangible steps that solidified my promise to myself to never, ever go back. If you follow these steps as I've outlined them here, you will have laid the foundation for your very own permanent transformation.

The Five Steps to Permanent Weight-Loss Transformation

Take "before" data. Until I stepped on the scale to get my starting weight for the weight-loss challenge, I had only an approximation of my actual weight. The last time I had weighed myself was when I was thirty-one and weighed 210 pounds—it had been ten years! I didn't own a scale or even a full-length mirror, but I knew I was heavier than ever before. I had worn a size 18 when I was 210 pounds, and I was now up to size 24. I estimated that being three sizes up made me 40–60 pounds heavier. I told myself I didn't need a scale because I *knew* I was at my heaviest.

When I finally stepped on the scale, I was surprised at the relief I felt— first when I realized it read 250 and not 350, as I'd originally misread, and second, because identifying my starting point gave me the power to begin moving forward. Knowing this number also freed up my mental focus; instead of guessing and wondering where my weight was, I now had a clear marker of where I stood.

At my heaviest, I did everything I could to avoid being in pictures, but looking back now at the pictures I do have is rewarding and validating. It reminds me of how far I've come—it's something I'm extremely proud of. To this day, I'm still finding random photos from that time that I've stashed away, and they never fail to reinforce my motivation.

It's Your Turn: Take the first empowering step by getting on the scale and documenting your starting weight. Make the promise to never see that number again. Then, snap a before photo, or find a recent picture that captures the current shape of your body. File this image away as just a bit of historical data—don't hang it around your neck or torture yourself with self-loathing. If you want, take a new picture every week or two, but don't feel the need to analyze it or use it to make judgments, positive or negative. Always reflect and act from a place of pride about who you are today and who you'll become in the future.

Define "how." In my case, the "how" started with getting into the rhythm of preparing my own meals and taking a daily walk. I drastically altered my relationship with food, eating only meals that I made for myself, which empowered me with the ability to control the number of calories I was eating.

For exercise, I knew that, at my weight, the first thing I had to do was walk (this was before I knew about kettlebells). The day after I weighed in for the contest, I woke up at six A.M. and drove over to a local trail that had a two-mile loop. Every day—and I mean every single day—I walked that two-mile trail, and one day a week I looped around twice, making the total distance four miles. It wasn't easy—my lower back was killing me, but I pushed through because I had a greater purpose: to renew my life.

I walked almost daily for years, even after I started training with kettlebells. I wasn't walking to burn calories, but to continue to strengthen my connection with the power and confidence of my physical body. I think this is something a lot of us, especially women, lose touch with—we forget how capable and strong our bodies are and how invigorated and dynamic they can, and want, to be.

It wasn't until I picked up the kettlebell that I began to see the real potential begin to show in my body. If walking was the spark, the swing was the fire. Just a few weeks after I started swinging the kettlebell in my garage, the muscles on my body began to show tone—my beautiful shape and strength was building up from the inside out.

I was so inspired by my rapid results, I emerged from my garage a kettlebell evangelist—I started taking my kettlebell to the park or the track, where I'd warm up with a walk and then get into my swings. I would show off a little to people who had never seen a kettlebell, much less knew what to do with one. I would take my kettlebell inside the house and swing in the kitchen between washing dishes and basting a turkey. The swing became a part of my life—not something separate from it—unlike other exercises I had tried in the past. I couldn't come up with a valid excuse not to do it. My workouts provided visible results fast by burning fat and building muscle, never took me more than thirty minutes, made me feel strong and powerful, and helped me realize that my body really was made to move. It was a revelation.

It's Your Turn: Order your kettlebell, and while you wait for it to arrive, start walking. Walk today for ten minutes. Then do it again tomorrow for twenty minutes, and work toward being able to walk one to two miles, four to five times a week. Walking outside is best, but if all you can get to is a treadmill, jump on it.

When you get your kettlebell, see page 85 to learn how to swing and begin your workouts. The swing will help you build strength and endurance, improve flexibility, and promote rapid weight loss. Pick up the bell and start swinging, and swing at least twice a week for twenty to thirty minutes, and you will makeover your body in a way you never thought possible.

Your first step with food is to take an honest look at what you're eating each day—what are the triggers that drive you to overeat? It may not be about eating an excess of junk food, like it was for me. It could be stress eating, snacking, or meal skipping (which creates binge eating), or a combination of all of these habits. To step away from any behaviors that drive unconscious eating, get grounded by working on your cooking skills. Don't worry if you aren't too familiar with your kitchen—when I changed my diet and starting cooking for myself, I had never roasted a chicken, grilled a steak, or made a pot of soup, so I know exactly where you might be coming from. If you want to make a great investment in your health, look for a local cooking class to take, which is what I did in the beginning. Also be sure to check out Part Three, where you'll find a full breakdown of the Swing Diet, along with basic tips and recipes that will help make eating right easy.

Establish your "why." On the very first day I started walking, I knew I was saving my life. That's how deeply I knew that what I was doing was right. Out there in the fresh air, I began reconnecting with my physical body, and I started an inner dialogue to help create a stronger connection. Since I was convinced my heart was in terrible shape, I focused my attention there, and with each step I imagined the grateful comments my heart would be saying to me if it had a voice: "Thank you for melting this fat away from me"; "Thank you for not making me work so hard"; "I feel better and stronger every day"; "We're going to do this." As silly as it sounds, it helped me bring together my mind and body. I finally felt like every part of me had come together to achieve the goal of creating a new life.

Not all my reasons for transforming my body were so thoughtful or deep—I wanted to remove the fat from my body because of the physical burden it was causing, but I also wanted it gone so I could finally look great and feel sexy and confident. I wanted it all, and I knew I was finally going to get it.

It's Your Turn: Let's bring your motivation to life by describing it. Figure out what lights that fire for you, and own it. This commitment to change is all about you—don't look to others to define your motivation or to "borrow" a reason, because it won't last. So the question is: what do you want? Maybe you want to heal your body from the inside out and give yourself the gift of health. Or you want to feel attractive and confident, to be able to try on clothes and feel great in them. Or you want to stop feeling depressed every time you catch a glimpse of yourself in the mirror or in a picture. Perhaps you want to get good at something, to create a skill that helps build your confidence in your abilities. I know learning how to swing and teaching myself how to cook were ground-level motivators for me, but they weren't the primary "why" that created the takeoff—for you, they might be just that. Motivation can come in many forms—find your why and take ownership of it.

Take the confidence challenge. There was a time when I would have believed that someone saw the Easter Bunny walking down the street before I believed that permanent weight loss was possible. But now here I sit with six years of maintenance under my belt—and not only can I say it's possible, I can say it's not that hard. When I started eating fewer calories and swinging the kettlebell, I started losing weight, and I continued to lose it until I created the body I wanted. Now I work to keep that body and to get stronger, not weaker, as I age.

All those years I wrestled back and forth with my weight, permanent weight loss was possible—I just didn't *believe* it was. I didn't have the confidence in my ability to make lasting changes. It was only when I acknowledged my own strength and ability to commit that I was able to change my life.

It's Your Turn: First off, remove the cloud of doubt or depression that's settled in over the topic of your weight—stop the doubts that start creeping in as soon as you start to consider changing your diet and exercise habits. There's nothing *bad* about making changes to improve your life—shift your perspective to see your commitments to swing your kettlebell and to eat right as gifts to yourself, because that's what they really are. I'm not smarter or luckier or more capable than anyone else, but I created permanent weight loss first by accepting that it was possible and believing it was not a myth. Permanent weight loss starts with the first pound, and if you can lose 1 pound then you can lose 100—the formula doesn't change, so stick with it and you will create the body you've always wanted.

Track your progress. The best thing about my weight loss was that it happened quickly. I started walking and preparing my own foods in January 2005, and four weeks later, I had lost 20 pounds. Then I lost 5 pounds a week for four straight weeks. After that, I lost 3 to 4 pounds a week, and in three months time, I had lost 50 total pounds, going from 250 to 200 pounds. In the next two months, I lost an additional 25 pounds at a rate of about 2 pounds a week, reaching a total of 75 pounds lost by the six-month anniversary of my starting date. By the end of November, I was 142 pounds—down 33 more. From November to April, I fine-tuned my body weight to 132 (another 10 pounds lost). Overall, I had lost 118 pounds in sixteen months. And through that entire period, I never hit a plateau—never! Every week I lost some amount of body weight.

I only weighed myself once a week until I got to my original goal weight of 142. At that point I knew that if I kept doing what I had been doing, it wouldn't be difficult to get to 132—10 more pounds after losing more than 100 pounds seemed like a drop in the bucket.

It's Your Turn: If you follow through on your commitment to consistency and you stay honest with yourself, you can *expect* results instead of just hoping for them. An important part of staying honest is

・・・

Your Goals Await

I know you have a dream weight in your head, and I've got a surprise for you—it's going to change! Your initial goal should be one that you can honestly strive for with everything in you, and let the momentum carry you forward from there. I discovered that once I created momentum it was easy to keep losing. Establish a timeline for your initial goal and then when, not if, you hit it, create your next goal (based on the success of meeting the first). As you begin to see your body's true potential, don't be afraid to let your ultimate goal evolve—be prepared to push through what you thought were your limits and redefine what it means to be your best.

・・・

tracking your progress, which includes writing down the foods you eat each day and monitoring your weight each week. I recommend only weighing yourself once a week until you get within striking distance of your goal weight. There are too many variables to take into consideration on a daily basis, but they even out over the course of a week. What I've learned from my husband, Mark, is the importance of a "trendline"— the path your progress would follow, typically up or down, if it were drawn on a chart. Whether it's your body weight or your training (are you getting stronger, leaner, more fit, and so on), moving in the right direction should be your focus.

For your workouts, be sure to use the workout journals (see pages 240–246), especially in the beginning as you focus on achieving an equal work-to-rest ratio—when your rest and workout times are the same. As your swing skills improve and you advance to the more complex workouts, use the logs to track your progress and to increase in reps. This way you'll know what number of reps created the best workout for you before and you'll be able to push yourself further next time. You'll create amazing progress when you ensure that each time you work out, you up the challenge just enough to push your body into the next level.

When you follow these five steps, you will be following in the footsteps of my own path to permanent weight loss. This path is based on proven methods for rapid body transformation: swinging a kettlebell at least twice a week and lowering your calories. It is impossible to completely change your eating and exercise habits and not lose weight. Do the work, make the changes, and the body will follow because it has to—you are in charge, so lead the way. The sooner you start creating these habits, the better—research has shown that maintaining weight loss actually gets easier over time. And I'll tell you it's the truth!

In This Together

I am still (and will forever be) on the path alongside you as you make a commitment to transform your body. I know what I'm capable of, and therefore I know what you are capable of. I'll always push to take myself further and to create continued progress in my life and my body—especially now that I know the possibilities. When you start swinging your kettlebell in your living room, I am in my garage training my butt off. When you are chopping cabbage for your salads, making tomato and vegetable soup, and packing your lunch, I am in my kitchen doing the same. You are not alone on this journey.

Now get ready to learn how to swing!

PART TWO

Body

6

Get the Body You Want in Less Time

In the twenty-five-plus years that the American Council on Exercise (ACE) has been around, it's seen plenty of fitness trends and has offered reviews of thousands of products, from the ones that seem like gag gifts to the genuine exercise tools. When the kettlebell started popping up on ACE's radar in 2005, thanks to the increase in use by personal trainers across the country, the calorie burn and workout efficiency claims were so outrageous, they had to invest in a study to see if they were true. Could people really do a complete workout in just twenty minutes? Could they really burn almost 300 calories in that time? Could they replace weights and cardio with just this one tool?

So they put some top science folks from the University of Wisconsin on the case. After conducting a research study, the researchers came back to ACE with answers. Here's a recap of what they said, in nonscientific terms: yes, yes, and yes. Or as Chad Schnettler, one of the researchers, put it: "For people who might not have a lot of time, and need to get in a workout as quickly as possible, kettlebells definitely provide that."

The Kettlebell Makes an Entrance

When I was first introduced to the kettlebell, I was skeptical—from what I could tell, it seemed just like any other type of dumbbell, and I had tried lifting weights in my twenties and never seen the results I wanted. But my husband, Mark, had fallen in love with the kettlebell and, like a kid with a new toy, kept encouraging me to try it. Mark had trained his body obsessively for decades with every type of weight and training method imaginable, but by 2003 the kettlebell had become the only tool used in his personal workouts—what was so special about this little, solid, single ball of cast iron?

Mark demonstrated how to do the swing, and I tried it—the motion felt natural and relatively easy, but I wasn't sold yet. All I found truly attractive about this new way of exercise was that I could do it in my garage, which meant I didn't have to set foot in a gym. Even though I had lost 50 pounds from changing my diet and walking, I was still heavy and didn't want to watch myself exercise in front of a mirror, let alone where other people watch me. Plus, the kettlebell was a form of weight-resistance exercise, which I knew I had to do to create muscle and tone; if I had any chance of looking good after losing the weight, I had to give my body some shape underneath all the fat.

My workouts started small—just a few sets of 10 reps with rest between each set. I wasn't working toward anything at first; I just wanted to get each workout over with. Within a couple weeks, I had worked up to 20 sets of 10 reps each. Then I taught myself the One-Hand Swing because I needed some variety. With the One-Hand Swing added to my repertoire, I started to focus more on workout patterns, rather than just total number of swings. It became a kind of game for me to piece workouts together—10 Two-Hand Swings, followed by 10 One-Hand Swings with my right arm, then 10 One-Hand Swings with my left arm, and so on. I was so distracted by the fun of creating the workouts that I didn't realize how much work I was actually doing. It was then that I saw myself in the dressing room mirror.

The History of the Kettlebell   By Mark Reifkind

The kettlebell was originally used in Russia, starting as far back as the year 1700, as a counterweight to measure grain. It was perfect for this process because the handle made it easier to place on and take off the scale. It soon became a measure of a peasant's strength, and all the eyes in the village were on the one who could lift it overhead in a variety of ways.

What started out as a simple test of strength soon evolved into an endurance contest with higher and higher repetitions being the goal. Swinging the bell, pressing it, and snatching it (swinging it in one movement overhead with one arm) became standard movements.

Centuries later the Soviets brought the kettlebell back as a training tool. They came to realize just how effective it was for building strength and endurance, and soon it became standard-issue training for their military, law enforcement, and Olympic athletes. It is still used to this day, which means this traditional, pre-industrial tool has a surprisingly practical application. Pavel Tsatsouline, chief instructor of the Russian Kettlebell Challenge (RKC) and the man who brought the kettlebell to our shores, calls the kettlebell "low tech, high concept."

The kettlebell's unique design, with the bulk of the weight offset from the handle, allows it to actually be swung as opposed to just lifted. This is the crucial difference between a kettlebell and a dumbbell. The dumbbell is essentially just an extension of your arm, but the kettlebell will revolve around in your hand, pivoting according to its own pathway.

The swinging motion is also what makes the kettlebell fun. I've never had anyone look over at me while I was leading him or her through a set of bicep curls and say, "I love this—this is fun!" And yet I hear that almost every time I teach someone how to swing a kettlebell.

It had been six weeks since I picked up the kettlebell and started swinging. I had done every workout in my garage with no mirrors, no clocks, just me and the kettlebell and my choreographed workouts. I didn't feel like I had been doing that much, but I was in for a big surprise.

While trying on clothes in the Target dressing room, I glanced at myself in the mirror and saw for the first time in my life, at the age of forty-one, the shoulder and arm development I had seen only on athletes' bodies. I couldn't believe it. Who was this person? She was a dream; she was the girl I always wanted to be. Suddenly, I saw the miracle, the possibilities right before my eyes. This epiphany changed the course of my journey. I wasn't going to settle anymore—I wanted it all: the muscle of an athlete, a silhouette I could feel great about, and the energy to push myself further than I ever imagined I was able to go.

The Right Kind of Resistance

The kettlebell is a form of weight-resistance training. Like strength training done with standard weights (dumbbells, barbells, and so on), it uses gravity to place a challenge on your muscles. As you lift a weight or swing a kettlebell through the air, gravity is trying to bring the weight back down to the ground—when you use your muscles to oppose this force, you demand your tissues get to work. And when muscles are worked, they break down and rebuild, and with each workout they become stronger, denser, more efficient calorie-burning machines. The kettlebell is one of the most effective forms of weight-resistance training because it operates on multiple planes—unlike traditional strength training, where the movements are static and fixed in nature, the kettlebell creates a dynamic movement that forces you to create and resist momentum. This engages and strengthens more muscle tissues at one time, which allows you to efficiently build fat-burning muscle and create beautiful tone faster than with other methods.

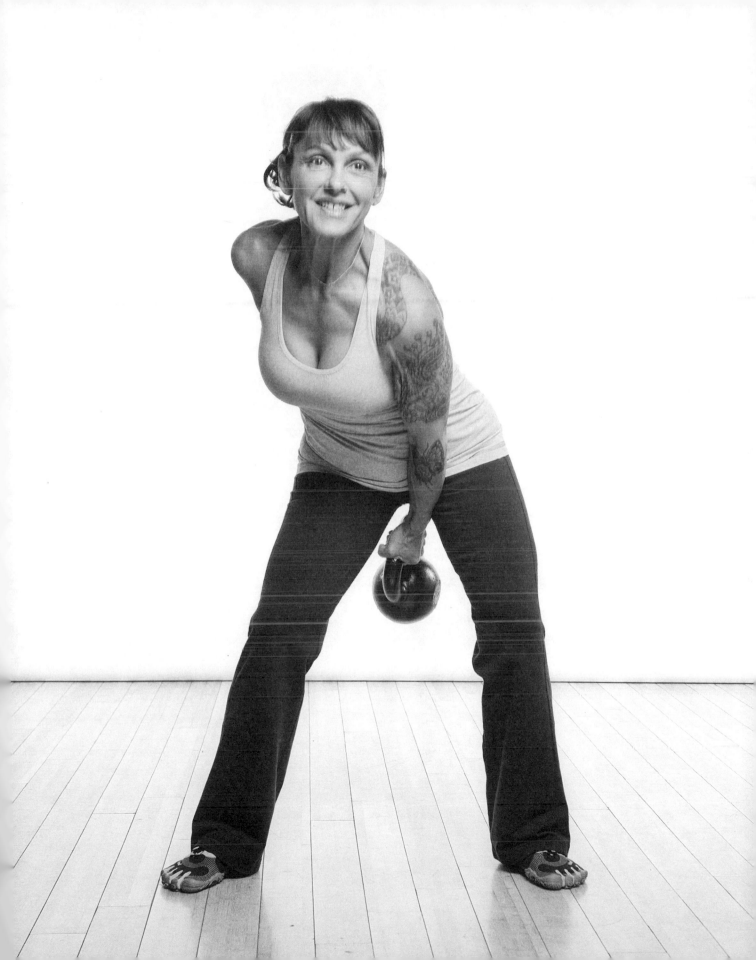

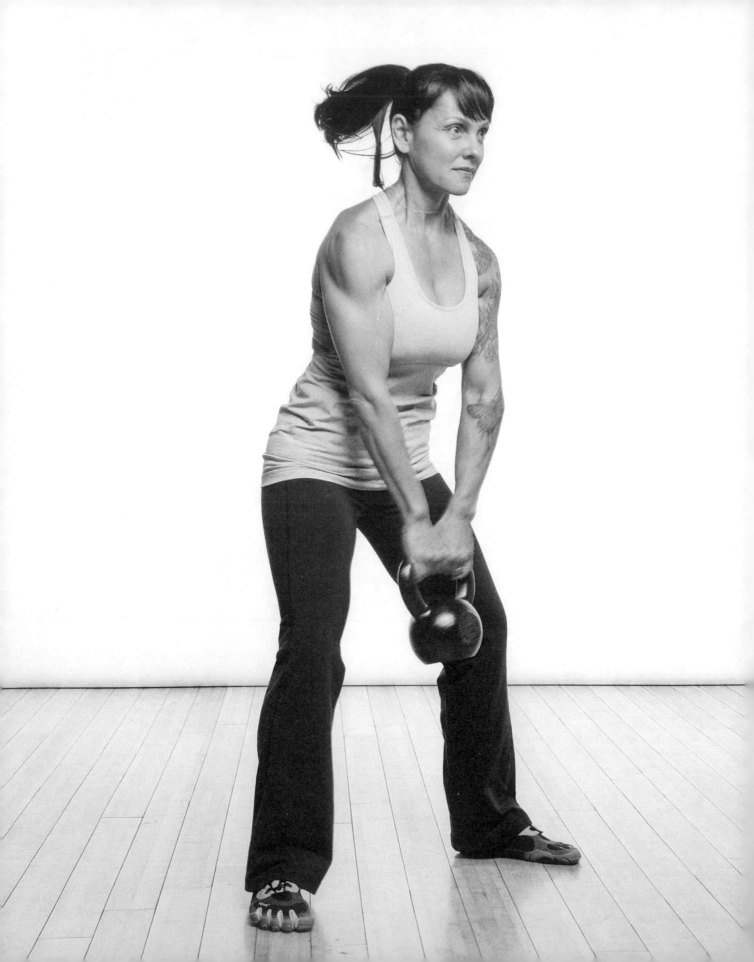

In that moment, the kettlebell gave me the hope that had evaded me in my past attempts at weight loss—it gave me an undeniable, visible sign that I was doing more than losing weight; I was transforming my body.

Over the next year, I diligently completed my kettlebell workouts and made my own meals. I created dozens of workouts that would push my body and demand progress from it—and my body responded with results, dropping weight consistently for sixteen months straight and revealing incredible muscle tone. Five years later, the swing is still redefining my expectations of my body, pushing me to get stronger and to increase muscle density, which makes my body more efficient at burning calories and using energy.

It was not by accident that my body transformed as a result of my kettlebell workouts. In fact, as I would eventually discover when I became a certified kettlebell instructor, the kettlebell is the best single apparatus for total body transformation. It wasn't that I got lucky; it's that the kettlebell works. Here's why the kettlebell enabled me to complete the journey and why it can do the same for you:

- **Whole Body Workouts:** The kettlebell can help you build strength and endurance, improve flexibility, and promote weight loss. It's an all-in-one, multifunctional, multitasking ball of wonder. There is simply no other single exercise method or tool that can change your body as completely or as quickly as the kettlebell.

- **No Bulk:** Typical strength-training exercises have you lift weights by body part—chest, back, legs, and so on. Guess what happens when you do that? You create chunky, snap-on body parts that seem to function individually rather than as parts of a whole. With the kettlebell, you focus on movements that engage your entire body as a unit, which is why the workouts will make you look athletic and toned, not bulky and brawny.

- **Easy on the Joints:** Your knees, ankles, and hips absorb the pressure of your weight when you do activities like walking, running, or jumping. If you're significantly overweight, the pressure from these kinds of activities can be especially taxing. Does that mean you won't ever be able to get a great cardio workout? Nope. Just grab a kettlebell, which allows you to get an awesome cardiovascular workout without the wear and tear on your joints. Hooray for no impact!

- **Hassle-Free:** You don't have to be coordinated or athletic to experience the benefits of a kettlebell, nor do you have to have a lot of money or special clothing or tools. It's simple, and it works without fail. Sometimes the simplest things can create the most profound change.

These benefits can be experienced to some degree from a variety of kettlebell movements, including exercises such as the deadlift, squat, clean/press, Get-Up, and the snatch. While you may have seen people attempt these exercises, you most likely have not seen them done correctly—they require advanced skills and really should only be done if you have very specific strength goals. It's important to master the swing first because it is the foundation to all other kettlebell exercises. It also has the greatest fat-burning potential; so if weight loss is your goal, look no further than the swing.

The Magic of the Swing

The swing takes all the benefits of the kettlebell and lifts it to a whole other level of greatness. Simply working out with kettlebells is not the same as training with the kettlebell swing. It would be like saying you've been to Las Vegas or Atlantic City when all you've done is bought a $1 lottery ticket at the corner store. In both cases, you might be playing the odds, but you have not had the *experience*. You have not seen the lights and the outrageousness, the spectacle of it all. *The swing is the experience.*

What creates the experience of the swing is the momentum, or the rhythm created by the motion. When you swing the kettlebell, you are moving it ballistically, which means that you are swinging the weight, not lifting it. Much like a bullet or missile, the kettlebell continues to move through space on its own after you've applied force to it. With the swing, you harness the power of momentum created by your hips as you put the bell into motion, and then the kettlebell moves upward on its own. You use your hips, legs, and thighs to create the movement, and your upper body comes along for the ride, keeping you tethered to the bell. The benefit is you can swing so much more weight than you can lift, and more weight means a greater challenge for your body, which translates to faster results.

How It Works

Let me tell you a little about why the swing is so incredibly effective at transforming your body. It all comes down to its ability to rapidly and thoroughly create muscle and muscle tone, which enables you to shape your body from the inside out. This process of shaping your body from the inside out all begins with contraction, which the swing generates throughout your body.

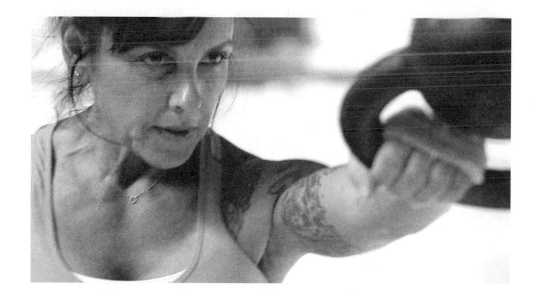

· ·

Why Women Should Learn to Love Muscle

*Muscle mass declines in both men and women as they age. It can
start as early as thirty, but once you turn fifty, you lose muscle at
a rate of 0.4 percent per year. For women, this can be especially
dangerous since women generally have less muscle on their bodies to
begin with. Add to that the fact that after menopause, decreasing
levels of estrogen leads to weakened bones, and you have a collision
of potentially devastating body changes that can lead to poor balance,
broken bones, and limited physical function. What's the most
prescribed solution to this health threat? Weight-resistance exercises
like the kettlebell swing. The sooner you start swinging that weight,
the more likely you are to build muscle. Lose weight, tone your body,
and help prevent the effects of aging.*

· ·

Your muscles function in a chain of action to reaction: contraction =
tension = tone = strength. When you contract a muscle, you create tension.
This tension, in turn, is what creates tone. The tone you want on your
arms, the sculpting you want of your abs, and the shape you'd like to see
on your legs—these all originate from the act of contraction which, like I
mentioned, happens all over your body when you train with the swing.
When muscular contractions are repeated and they become a skill
instead of just a reaction, you have created strength. And once your
muscles have strength, you have earned something worth preserving,
a precious attribute you are willing to work to keep—a precious asset
that also happens to look amazing in tank tops.

When muscles contract often, they stand ready to contract even when
they're at rest. Everyone has a resting level of tension in our muscles all
day. You've probably seen people who look muscular even when they're

doing nothing—these people have a higher resting level of tone in their muscles because they have been contracting them regularly; in other words, they've been working out to the point where their muscles at rest have shape. Even if they have a layer of fat over the muscle, you can distinguish trained bodies versus untrained bodies (it's so much more attractive to have some shape going on!).

There are three basic types of muscle contractions: raising weight (concentric contraction), lowering weight (eccentric contraction), and holding weight (isometric or static contraction). Swinging a kettlebell involves all three types of contraction at different points in the swing. When you are standing up with the bell, you are using concentric contraction; when the bell is lowering between your legs, this creates eccentric contraction; and when you are tethered to the bell as you hold your body steady while the bell swings to and fro, you are using isometric contraction.

When you combine all of these for each repetition, you experience a synergistic effect that very quickly creates spectacular results in muscle tone and strength. Then we add in the element of acceleration—the speed of the swing—and the effects are magnified even further. The loads that your muscles and your body are experiencing when you swing are five to ten times greater than the amount of weight on the face of the kettlebell. You simply can't create the same type of workout with a static lifting motion.

The better you get at the swing, the more force you can produce and the faster your results will be, which really can't be said for many other activities. Once you get past being a beginning runner, it's very hard to run faster. The same goes for swimming. In fact, the better you get at most cardiovascular activities, the fewer calories you burn and the fewer muscles you engage because your body gets so efficient at these movements. Keeping your heart rate up and keeping the muscles stimulated is very tough as you advance, unless you up the mileage and time spent training, which often leads to injuries.

You aren't going to experience any of these problems with the kettlebell swing. I'm going to teach you how to increase the workload and the workout *dramatically* by simply modifying your rest intervals or moving up to a slightly heavier kettlebell. Here's all you really need to know about the swing: nothing works all your muscles better or simultaneously burns more fat and builds more muscle. Nothing.

The Body Possible

The benefit of sculpting your internal musculature while you lose weight is that you create a body that has beautiful shape and definition. I want you to think of it as building up your inner mannequin that will look amazing in all your favorite clothes. If you don't add muscle while you lose weight, you end up with soft, loose skin that just hangs on your body like clothes on a wire hanger—in other words, you end up looking skinny and fat at the same time. But when you put those same clothes over a solid, shapely mannequin, you have a body and an outfit worth showing off.

That's how I managed to lose so much weight and not end up with the dreaded aftermath of saggy skin, a telltale sign of former obesity. The musculature I crafted with my swings allowed my skin to almost shrink-wrap back into shape. I can't tell you how many times I have been asked this question about loose skin. Complete strangers ask me this question all the time, and you know why? Because I look great and they can't believe I ever weighed close to 300 pounds.

I find the question very personal, but at the same time, it's a strange indicator of how unbelievable my results seem to people. Depending on how much weight you have to lose, you might experience it for yourself, and if you do, try to consider yourself lucky when a complete stranger asks you about your skin.

I'm not saying you'll be seeing me in a bikini anywhere, ever. I am close to fifty, I've had a couple of children, and I'm far from perfect compared to the perpetually young standards of today. What I can say, however, is that without a doubt I would not trade my body with anyone. I am not ashamed of any imperfections I may have, whether I perceive them as such or someone else does, and I especially couldn't care less about what anyone else thinks of my body.

You don't have to be enormously overweight, or overweight at all, to have concerns about loose or low-hanging skin, especially on your arms where your triceps should be. You may be able to hide it on your legs, but it gets hot in the summertime, and I know all women—and men too—want to be able to look and feel good in a tank top, especially if you're over forty.

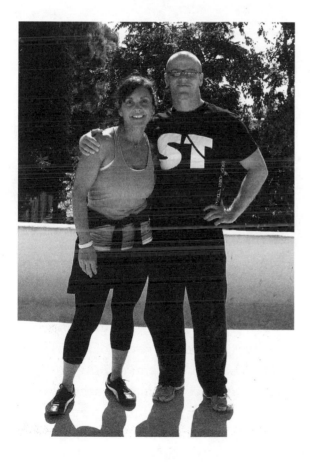

When I was first interviewed by Tim Ferriss for *The 4-Hour Body*, I talked about Michelle Obama's arms and how they were all the rage, especially among middle-aged women. Middle-aged women saw those arms and how she proudly displayed them, and they were envious of how confident and strong she looked. More than that, we were in awe because here was a woman who was over forty wearing sleeveless shirts, not just in her backyard but all over the country and in front of cameras. And she looked great doing it.

You know why her arms look amazing? Because she has muscle! Toned upper arms look marvelous because they have the shape of the musculature underneath. Building and activating the muscles of your arms is the first part of getting toned arms. To bring your muscles back to life, you must give them the job they were originally created to do: work. The second part of getting shapely arms is to get rid of the layer of fat that's covering up the beautiful muscle you're about to build. The kettlebell swing will take care of both of these tasks simultaneously.

Since the power and momentum of the kettlebell swing is generated with a hip and leg movement, you might think there would be no advantage for your upper body. In reality, the swing will fire up and engage just about every muscle in your body, from toes to nose. Some of the less obvious muscular contractions happening when you swing are in the lat (back) muscles, the abdominal muscles (from breathing), the triceps and biceps, and the pectorals (chest). You will be using a lot of muscle without even knowing it, but your body knows, and the effects will be obvious as they begin to remodel your shape and show up in your mirror.

The Beauty of Expansion

The swing will open you up to face the world with absolute confidence and vitality. You'll discover that it's an empowering move based on expansion, a movement that literally opens you up to life. It will broaden your chest, pull your shoulders back and open, and strengthen your back. The swing is the solution to the seated existence in which your daily activities have made you barely strong enough to oppose gravity. Think about it—how much of your day do you just sit while engaged in other activities? Working on a computer, driving, reading, eating, watching TV . . . all sitting activities.

All these activities combine to create a closed-off posture with all forces pulling inward—you've seen the people (maybe you're one of them) with forward sloping, rounded shoulders. This is more than an outward appearance; these are physical signs that reflect an internal attitude of defeat. You simply cannot feel your strongest, most confident, and most beautiful self when your body is physically closing in around you, shutting you off from the world. The swing will help you fight back

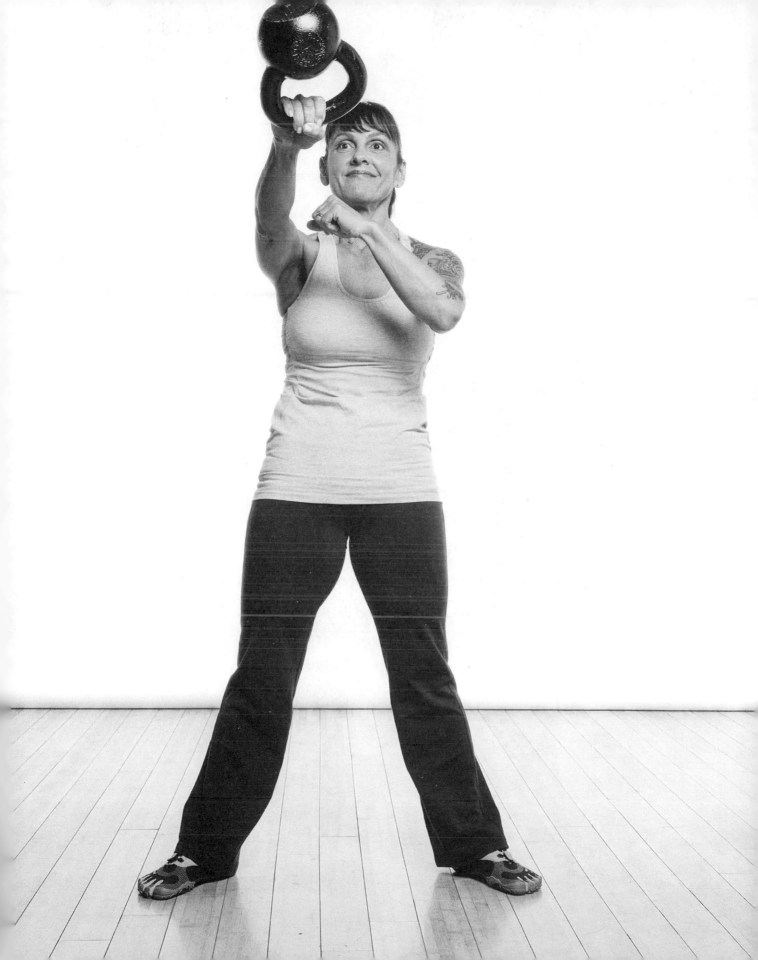

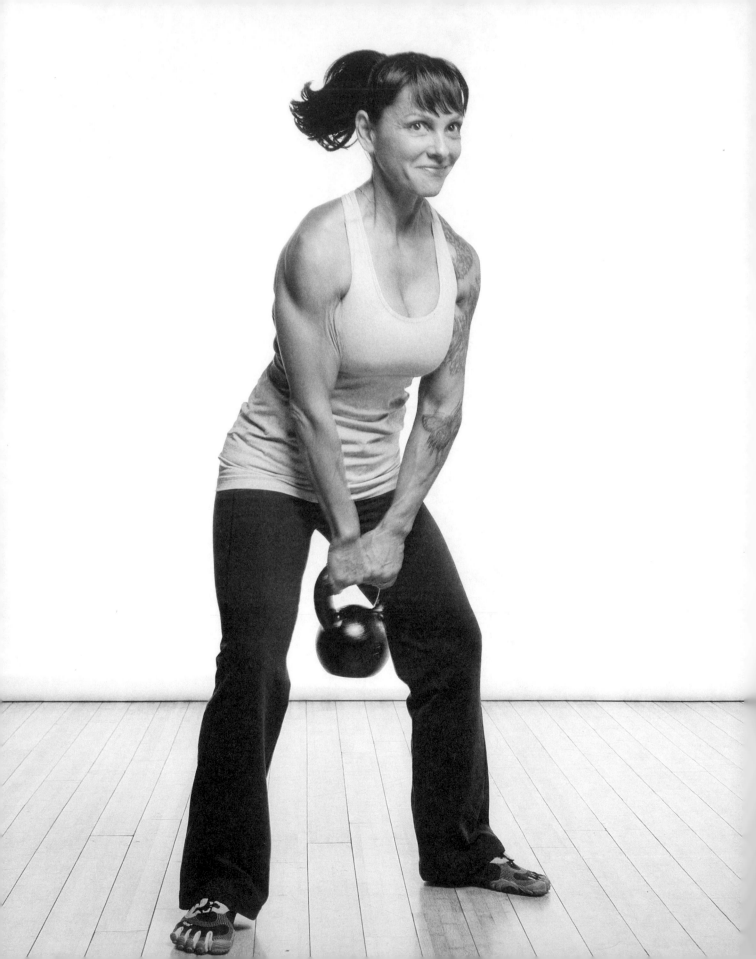

against the forces that shrink your energy and enthusiasm for life. When you try it, you'll understand: it feels celebratory and expansive. As you begin to swing, focus on this quality of the movement—see your body opening up, your confidence and energy growing. Get ready to take on life with a renewed sense of strength and the power to overcome anything that comes your way.

No Room for Excuses

The kettlebell swing helped me realize how little I needed to be my best. With one movement and one bell, I created the best version of myself, and it all started the day I walked into our garage gym and picked up the kettlebell. The garage was dark and dusty and filled with a lot of my husband's power-lifting gear, but what I experienced in that room was a bright and hopeful revelation. It was there that I realized I was in charge of creating my own change; that I could accomplish anything I wanted, and that included creating the body of my dreams.

I never thought it was possible for me to experience life from a place where I feel connected to my confidence, where I feel truly strong of body and mind, but I am proof that it is possible.

As you get ready to swing, I want you to think about stripping away all the junk in your life—all the baggage, blame, crappy foods, failed attempts at fitness, messy emotions. Trust yourself enough to accept an end to the fight between you and your body and to adopt a new mantra: it's not that hard. Eat real foods, swing a kettlebell, and repeat. See yourself walking into a room where it's just you and this little bell of cast iron—can you pick it up and transform your life? Yes, you can, and it's that simple. You're going to have to work really hard to find an excuse. You can think about it some more while I get back to swinging.

7 Getting Ready to Swing

To get started with the swing, here's what you need: nothing. That's right—you can actually start practicing the swing movement with just your body. I call these Air Swings, and they will familiarize you with the motion and even provide a challenging workout for some of you. Of course, you should get a kettlebell as soon as possible, but don't let that wait time go to waste—see page 96 to learn how to perform an Air Swing.

Throughout the rest of this chapter, I'm going to give you some instructions for selecting your kettlebell, along with some information on other products you can pick up *after* you've started your workouts. Most of these are simple tools that can help your workouts, but they aren't all essential. Let's get to the most important tool first: the kettlebell.

Selecting Your Kettlebell

Because kettlebells are of European origin, they are usually sold in kilograms. One kilogram is equal to 2.2 pounds. The most common starting weights for a female are either an 8-kilogram or 12-kilogram kettlebell, which translates into 18 or 26 pounds. For a male, a good starting weight is 16 kilograms, which is 36 pounds. If you're a man over 200 pounds and/or you have experience weight training, then your starting kettlebell could be 20 kilograms (44 pounds).

The Two-Hand Swing is the exercise I will be putting most emphasis on in this book. With this movement, it's important to get a bell that's heavy enough—a bell that's too light may not give you the feedback you need to feel the proper motion. That being said, you can still get quite a workout using the swing movements with no weight. It's the movement itself that is so powerful, but when you add weight to it, it really becomes magic.

The drills in the Learn section (see pages 86–105) will teach you how to get into the correct positions and postures before adding weight to your workout. You will quickly become aware of how even a workout using just air can be more dynamic than almost anything else you've tried.

If and when you want to incorporate the One-Hand Swing, I recommend using a lighter kettlebell: 6 to 8 kilograms for women and 12 to 14 kilograms for men. If you are a female beginner, do not attempt the One-Hand Swing with anything over 10 kilograms; a male beginner should not attempt it with anything over 16 kilograms.

Somewhere Between a Dungeon and a Dream Factory

Personally, I like the no-frills approach to a workout space. It may result from being around so many serious, competitive lifters (including the one I've been married to for over twenty years), but I've learned that the most important detail in a workout space besides equipment is some hard rock music. This works for me because I find there's something about that atmosphere that says, "It's just me against the world"—and that makes me want to work hard. Certainly, I can see the appeal of more comfortable surroundings, especially a space that includes the luxury of heat. Swinging out in my garage in the winter (even in California) can get as cold as 32 degrees, but with bare feet and a frozen kettlebell handle, it's still never stopped me.

I know a lot of my clients and students prefer to swing in private, away from the eyes of family members who might be thinking, "That looks crazy!" The good news is, wherever you can carve out a space of four feet by six feet, you can swing a kettlebell. Add whatever you want to your space—claim it as yours with things that motivate you.

When you get to your workouts, make sure that small children and pets are not in the way, and for obvious reasons, do not swing in front of the TV. If you drop a bell, it shouldn't travel far, but how far it goes really depends on when you lose your grip during the motion of the swing. I have dropped a bell only a few times, only while I was moving it from one hand to another and mostly because I created too much power with my hips using a bell that was too light. I've never dropped a bell using the two-hand method, and most likely you won't either, but be smart about your surroundings.

Tools for Swinging

The first piece of additional equipment I recommend you have nearby is a clock with a second hand. The alarm clock I use is so old I don't even remember when I got it. The important part is not its age or its size—it's all about the second hand. I've since upgraded to a wall clock, but in all honesty, I still use both in my garage gym.

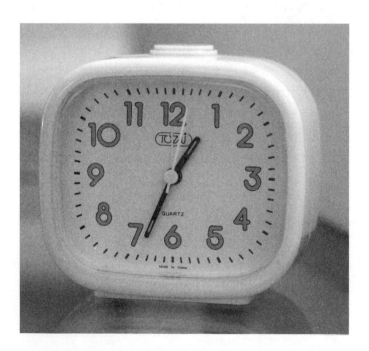

You'll need the second hand because establishing the pace of the swing is one of your first lessons, and the pace is one of the most important factors for your body to get when you start to practice and train with the swing. Eventually you will need to know the time of your sets (the number of swing reps before rest is taken) and the time of your rest periods, but we'll get to that later.

As you work your way up to progressions, you can also pick up a useful tool called an interval timer.

The most popular one I know of is called the Gymboss, and it is relatively inexpensive. You can also try to find an application for an interval timer on your smartphone, if you have one. The interval timer is helpful to me because it keeps track of how many total interval sets I've completed. At the same time, knowing the total time of a workout is the only way I know when to stop training. I'm sure my students appreciate this too.

Like I mentioned, I prefer to put on some rock music for my personal workouts, and I also use the same type of music for my advanced classes. I've trained plenty in silence, but I prefer motivating rhythms and lyrics. For my beginner-level classes, I put on dance music or upbeat pop songs. It's definitely a matter of taste, but I suggest picking something up-tempo to get you motivated for your workouts.

You should always have some water nearby. Water is a must, and it doesn't hurt to have a towel and some tissues on hand. If you have hardwood floors like I do, then I suggest lying down a simple doormat (I purchased mine at Ikea for a few bucks) to protect the floor. A fan is a luxury, although it can become a necessity in the summertime. Personally, I like sweating because it lets me know how hard I'm working—and I know I'm having a really good workout when my shins start to sweat.

When it comes to protecting your hands (if you care to do so—it's not required), weightlifting gloves are typically not recommended because the leather palms do not let the bell pivot in your hand, but many of my students use them. I've also seen people use cotton gardening gloves with the fingers cut off. My favorite option is my own creation: Tracy Rif's Sock Sleeves. I came up with the idea for Sock Sleeves out of necessity because gloves didn't work for me; I needed a fabric that was slippery and would allow smooth swings. I tried wristbands, but they were too thick. So I cut off the top of a sock—the part that goes around your ankle—and placed it around my palms, and voilà, problem solved. This inexpensive, yet effective solution has even been adopted at RKC Certifications and suggested in the RKC manual.

If you've ever spent much time in a gym, you've noticed there are mirrors all over the place. They're not just there to make you feel uncomfortable or for purposes of vanity; a mirror can be an invaluable tool when it comes to checking form. When training with the kettlebell, the only time you should use a mirror is when you encounter a mistake you can't feel your way out of (you can also use a video camera to see where any corrections need to be made). Usually you can feel when and how you're out of position, but identifying which specific part of the movement you are out of position on can be difficult, which is when a mirror can be helpful.

I don't, however, suggest a mirror for learning the swing because it tends to pull you forward and it delays the real feedback from your body. It takes too long for you to see your image and then transport the correction back to your brain. Imagine trying to learn to ride a bike while looking at your image in a mirror—there would be too many little movements trying to capture your vision. Instead, you want to refine your proprioception skills, to know where your body is in space. Once you've felt how to swing the right way, you'll be able to perceive where adjustments need to be made if a movement feels off.

I never teach anyone how to move the bell from two hands to one, or from one hand to another, in front of a mirror because they tend to look at the bell in the mirror, not at the one in their hands. Remember this when you begin to practice the One-Hand Swing and transfers—it's better to let your body become familiar with these exercises before you add in a mirror to improve or self-correct your form.

What to Wear

Here's what to wear when doing your kettlebell workouts: whatever is comfortable. Don't go out and buy anything special because it's not going to fit you for long. I trained in my jeans for years for exactly this reason. Unless some new clothes will fuel motivation, there is no practical reason to get them.

I knew I was going to lose 100 pounds, and that meant going from a size 24 to a size 8. I did not buy anything new until my clothes were literally falling off my body. Because I lost weight so quickly, I went from a size 24 to a 14, then down to a 10, then to a 6, never buying sizes in between. It would have only been a waste of money for me to buy clothes for those in-between sizes—that's how certain I was of where I was going, and I wasn't about to stop midway to my destination.

I wore jeans for almost three years of weight loss and workouts. The attire also lent itself to my hardcore approach and attitude; it was like an act of rebellion to refuse to go out and buy what other people said were appropriate exercise clothes. I really disliked the pretentiousness of all the skinny little "chickie-dos" (my mother's word) running around in their workout clothes or their tennis outfits . . . I did not want to be like them. I have to admit I recently started to wear exercise clothes because I found a brand called Lululemon, and the design and quality is attractive to me. I guess I've become a chickie-do, but I worked extremely hard to be able to feel great in the clothes that cling to my body.

When it comes to footwear for your workouts, you should wear a pair of flat-bottomed shoes, like Converse Chuck Taylors, Vibram FiveFingers (what I'm wearing in the pictures in this book), or something similar. Other common flat-soled shoes used by kettlebell athletes these days are made by brands like Puma and Merrell. Your feet are the connection to the ground, and you want to be solidly rooted to the ground when you're swinging. Soft, cushy shoes delay the feedback from the ground to your body. And every inch of heel height pushes your body forward 15 degrees, which disturbs your center of balance. For this reason, any kind of shoe with an incline is not recommended. No running shoes!

I prefer to train barefoot now, but that wasn't always the case. When I was fat, I never went barefoot because my feet were too weak to support my body. I wore shoes all the time, even indoors while doing housework because although I couldn't explain it at the time, my feet just weren't strong enough to handle the extreme load of my body weight, even while doing everyday tasks.

When you begin your workouts, I recommend you stick with flat-bottomed shoes, but as you progress, don't be afraid to try going barefoot down the road—it's liberating and lets you really feel the ground.

Eating Before and After Workouts

I train in the morning because I'm a morning person. I've trained as early as five thirty to get my workout in on days when I have other appointments or commitments that may interfere. I would train at three A.M. if I had to, but that's me.

Since I train first thing in the morning, I never eat beforehand. If you eat first, or give your body fuel as soon as you wake up, it has no reason to tap into stored energy because you've increased your blood sugar and your body will use what's immediately within reach. You want to train your body to go into its stored energy source—the fat. By exercising in a fasted state, you accelerate your body's ability to burn fat. Tapping into fat reserves will accelerate your weight loss, and it will help you develop the hormones necessary to burn fat by keeping your insulin levels low. Keeping insulin low is good for a number of reasons: it increases your ability to burn fat, decreases inflammation, staves off hunger, and keeps insulin sensitivity high, which reduces your chances of creating metabolic syndrome (the precursor to diabetes).

The other benefit of exercising in a fasted state is that you keep all the blood ready to surge into your muscles with energy and oxygen. If you are digesting food, the blood has to go to the stomach, which makes it unavailable to your muscles. It may take awhile to adapt to exercising in a fasted state, but you will and you'll realize how much better you feel during your workouts.

If you absolutely feel you have to eat before a workout, then it should be something small and easily digestible; something not too heavy in proteins, fats, or fiber because they take a long time to digest. Fruit is a good choice, or yogurt, or—and this is the only time you will hear me say this—half an energy bar would work too. If you opt for fruit, I recommend either melon or some slices of an apple.

When you are *not* jumping right into a workout, the rules for your morning meal swap—skip sugary options and go for a lighter protein like nuts.

If you have to train in the evenings before dinner, avoid eating a big meal at least two hours prior to your workout. Save your biggest meal for after your workout.

Remember, not eating forces your body to go into stored energy. To give you an idea of how much stored energy you have on your body, here are a couple quick examples: if you are 50 pounds overweight, you have 175,000 calories of stored energy; 30 pounds overweight means 105,000 calories of stored energy. You can afford to burn some of those reserves!

Once you've finished your workout, don't think of yourself as having earned the reward of food. For optimal weight loss, you should wait at least one hour and then eat a wholesome, balanced meal. If you wait awhile after training, your body will continue to tap in to fat stores.

An Active Warm-Up

I prefer the active warm-up of walking to a static warm-up of stretching. A 10-minute walk is just enough to get some blood pumping through my veins and to raise my body temperature, easing me into the more demanding kettlebell workout ahead. Mentally, I can clear my mind and separate my workout from the rest of my day.

That doesn't mean you shouldn't incorporate regular stretching into your life—creating and maintaining flexibility can be extremely important, especially as you get older. The difficult part about stretching, for me, is following through with it on a regular basis, but it's probably just because I don't like to sit still for long. There is a correct way to stretch, and it can be a learned skill just like any other physical activity. Being married to a former elite gymnast, I know firsthand the importance of stretching properly. I highly suggest working with someone who can show you how to stretch correctly if you want to use this as your warm-up. First thing's first, though—let's get some of this extra weight off, and then you can focus on improving your flexibility.

Scheduling Workouts

Your very first swing workout may be with no bell, but bell or no bell, you should not spend more than fifteen to twenty minutes practicing this new movement. You will be stretching and loading muscles you haven't felt for years, and regardless of any added weight, you will most likely experience soreness ranging from mild to significant discomfort when walking or sitting. Don't be scared of soreness; think of it as something you've earned thanks to your hard work, and remember it will go away (I recommend light stretching to help ease soreness). That being said, don't overdo it with the amount of time you spend swinging in the beginning. My Learn to Swing classes are never more than thirty minutes long, and this includes a lot of talking through instructions and exercise drills—the actual swing time is less than half that.

Once you are comfortable in establishing correct form and movement, your workouts will require no more than twenty to thirty minutes of your time, two to three days a week. You're not going to spend twenty to thirty minutes swinging nonstop; this is total time of your workouts, including rest periods. Aim to work out at least two days a week, but I think you'll be surprised to discover that you want more. Just be sure you give your body a day between workouts for recovery, practicing every other day at the most. Recovery is extremely important for progress because it's when your body makes physical changes or creates results—it doesn't happen when you're training. Training is the stimulation, and recovery is the adaptation.

"Can I Swing Every Day?"

Believe it or not, "Can I swing every day?" is one of the most common questions I hear. My reply is always the same: "If you could, I would be doing it right now." In fact, one of the reasons why I took up yoga was because I knew I shouldn't swing every day.

Let the swings do their best work by ensuring you give your body enough rest. If you feel you have to do something to accelerate your results, spend any free time you have on preparing foods and eating better, and walking to help improve your base level of fitness. If you like extra time, you're going to love the swing. Just twenty to thirty minutes, two times a week, spent swinging will leave you plenty of time to spend doing other activities that are important for your body and your life.

The most important point when it comes to scheduling your workouts is to establish a consistent time on your weekly calendar. Just as you take your kids to school at a certain time or you have that weekly work meeting, you have to get a regular time set for your workouts. I like to say, "If your plan is to not plan, then you don't have a plan." Having a plan is less about being strict and rigid and more about removing the problem of too much choice, which inevitably leads to procrastination.

If you have been using the excuse of having no time to workout, then I want you to take a bit more responsibility and replace, "I don't have time," with, "I won't make time," because that's what it really comes down to. What if you developed an illness or condition that required multiple doctors' appointments or, God forbid, hospitalization? Do you have the time for that? Or what if a family member did, would you not have time to take him to his appointments? Somehow we find time when tragedy strikes. Perhaps that's a bit dramatic, but I think you can either make the choice of how you spend your time now, or you can wait until something makes the choice for you. It's up to you.

I like to think of my choice to train as a reward, not a punishment or a do-or-die situation. I get to spend twenty to thirty minutes, two to three times a week, swinging a kettlebell, and in return I am rewarded with the priceless gift of a fit, healthy, toned, and capable body. If you cannot make time for it, then I'm not going to beg you to workout. Nobody has to beg me; in fact, nothing or no one could stop me from getting my workouts in each week. I'm showing you where the pot of gold is; if you don't want it, then don't cry about being poor. You can have the body you want; you can live a strong, healthy, active life. You can go through a personal transformation as incredible as mine—stop settling and start becoming the person you were meant to be.

Exercising for the Right Reasons

I want you to keep something in mind as you begin your workouts: think about swings as something you're doing to create a skill, not something you're doing to make up for the food you're eating. If progress is not the reason for training, and instead you're just trying to burn off extra calories, then you may be exercising for the wrong reasons. You may be putting in what are known as junk miles— workouts completed to make up for a poor diet, instead of done with the intention to create progress or results.

Will more exercise burn more calories? Yes, because it all comes back to science. That doesn't mean, however, that you'll create better or faster results. The return on the investment is minimal at best. I prefer to look at my exercise the way an athlete looks at his chosen sport. I ask myself: Am I getting better? Stronger? Leaner? Faster? Asking yourself these questions as you make progress will help you establish built-in markers of motivation. If you're simply spinning your wheels with no plan or thought to the progressive improvement of performance, then you're on a road to nowhere.

The Chance You Deserve

I'd like to say, "Give the swing the chance it deserves," but really it's about what you deserve—the swing is already secure in its greatness, it's yours that we are going to bring to life. As you begin with the swing, keep in mind that as with every new skill there is a learning curve— don't get discouraged because what you might lack in skill or talent, you can make up for in consistency. No matter your athletic (or nonathletic) history, you will begin to feel truly in charge of the movement after just 3-4 practices. You will also feel great improvements in your strength and cardiovascular health and see your body changing faster than you ever thought possible. Remember to feel the motion, rather than spend too much time thinking about it—like a kid on a swing, enjoy the rhythm and just have fun!

Learning the Kettlebell Swing

I've designed a system that will let you jump into your kettlebell training with confidence and will create results as quickly and safely as possible. The movements you are going to perform couldn't be simpler—they are based on the primal movement of the swing, which is a natural, fun movement that truly feels fabulous.

The LPT Best Body Plan

Even though the actual movements are simple, it's important to establish a foundational understanding of form, breathing, and rhythm. That's why I created the Learn, Practice, Train (LPT) Best Body Plan. **Learn, Practice,** and **Train** each represent a distinct phase that I will lead you through as you progress in your kettlebell workouts. Here's a quick preview of what you'll discover in each section:

- **Learn:** This phase will set the groundwork for your workouts and will show you how to maximize its effects from day one. I will also cover how to create your ideal workout with proper form and breathing, and tell you how to set up a great workout space. Remember—no gym required!

- **Practice:** This is when you'll first start to use a practice strategy I call On the Minute training. This is a basic method that will help you establish an understanding of intervals and a work-to-rest ratio—the amount of time you spend swinging to the amount of time you spend resting.

- **Train:** Once you reach this phase, you've already created outstanding changes in your body—now it's time to use advanced choreographed routines to continue pushing and improving your body. We'll also add in a few more moves in this phase.

And now, let's jump right in and get you swinging!

The Learn Phase

Since we're going to focus on one central movement—the Two-Hand Swing—I want you to have access to everything there is to know about the movement. It's not complicated or advanced, but creating a connection to all the parts of your body that come to life in the swing will reward you with better results. In the *Learn* part of LPT, you will become a true student of the swing—this will be your own personal training session with me as I guide you through basic drills to help you get the feel of the movement.

When you first learn how to swing, it's important to have an awareness of your spine and its formation, specifically the four natural curves that make it functional and allow you to create a straight spine. You may have heard the phrase *straight spine* before, but chances are, you don't really know what it is, how it feels, or what it looks like. A straight spine aligns the four natural curves that run from your neck down to your tailbone. When you start to work out with your kettlebell, keeping these four curves in mind will help protect your back:

The **cervical curve** includes the vertebrae that support your neck.

The **thoracic spine** makes up the middle back and represents the longest part of your spine.

The **lumbar** includes the thickest vertebrae (think of the foundation of a building) and is located in your lower back.

The **sacral curve** is where the bones at the base of your spine connect with your pelvic bone.

Even without the kettlebell, having an awareness of these important points along your spine can improve your general posture, help you breathe easier by opening up your airways, and enhance confidence— try it right now. Sit up straight, take a nice, strong inhale, and then exhale. See what I mean? An open, expanded chest and an upright posture can make you feel powerful and ready to take on life.

One misconception about creating a straight back is that you have to be upright to do it. In reality, you can actually be leaning forward and still have a straight spine, and this is the position you are going to create in your swings. As I break down the form of the swing for you, you'll learn the techniques to maintain a straight spine as you hinge through the motion.

It's Not a Squat (or a Front Raise)

I want to make an important distinction about the main movement for the swing: it's a hinge, not a squat, and you move the bell with the power of your hips, not by raising it with your arms. When people first see the swing and try to re-create the movement, they often go into a squat—for some reason it's the way their brains communicate the movement to their bodies. The problem is, if you just do a squat with the kettlebell, you're missing the most powerful and fun part of the swing. A squat is an up-and-down movement; a hinge allows you to swing back and forth.

When you squat (see "Incorrect" image, opposite page), your knees bend and move forward (many times past your toes, even though this isn't proper form) as you move up and down while staying vertical. Hinging originates from the point where your legs meet your torso. When you hinge (see "Correct" image, opposite page), you lean forward and push your butt backward while keeping your shins vertical. This creates a back-and-forth rocking motion, instead of an up-and-down one.

1

2

You also want to pay attention to your arms and shoulders. Don't try to lift the bell in front of you with your arms, instead let your hips drive the movement and create the momentum. Trust me, your arms are going to get plenty of work, but your hips are much stronger, so let them lead.

The other common mistake people make is thinking that the start of the swing happens in front, when really, just as a child on a playground backs up first to swing, you must back up the bell (it's often called a hiking motion), load your hips, and then create the swing.

I'm going to take you through some drills to help you get the feel of the swing movement.

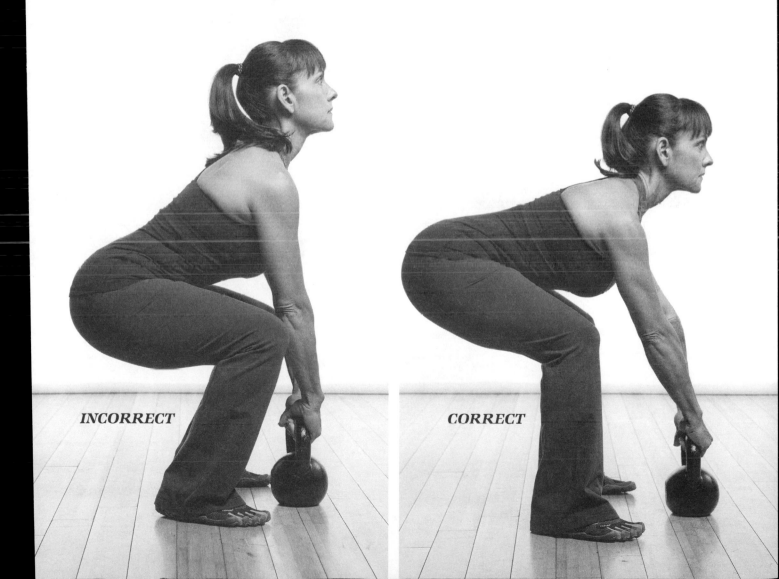

INCORRECT   **CORRECT**

The Chair Hinge Drill

Grab a standard four-legged chair and your kettlebell; place them two to three feet from one another. Stand with the back of your legs touching the chair, then step out about six inches and plant your feet slightly wider than hip-distance apart. You should be midway between the chair and the kettlebell. (If you don't have a kettlebell yet, there are several options to use as a placeholder: an empty milk container, an empty or half-full gallon of paint, a small pot, or even just a purse or backpack.)

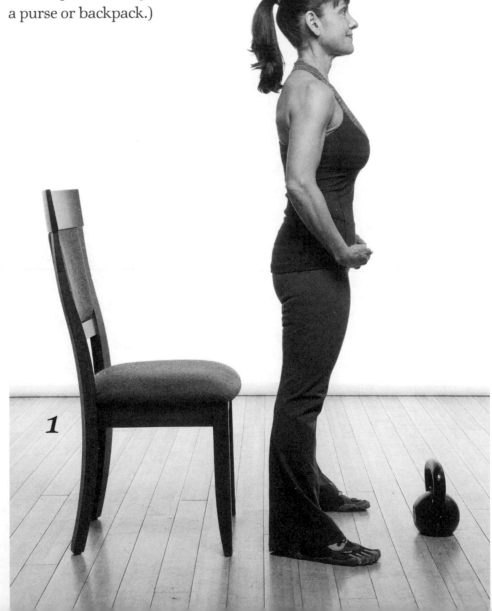

1

While keeping your back straight, hinge toward the chair behind you with your hands in the creases of your hips, pushing yourself backward (gently). As you perform this movement, visualize hinging back and down *as if* you were going to sit in the chair, but don't sit down. Feel your hamstrings and glutes stretch and load as you reach back with your butt, and then stand up.

As you stand up, contract your quadriceps muscles by lifting up on your kneecaps, and squeeze your glutes tightly. By doing this, you ensure that your legs are straight and your hips are forward. This is the top position of the kettlebell swing.

Repeat this same motion 5–10 times, only this time inhale as you hinge back and down, then sharply exhale as you stand up straight. The sharp exhalation at the top of the movement will create the inhalation for the next swing rep.

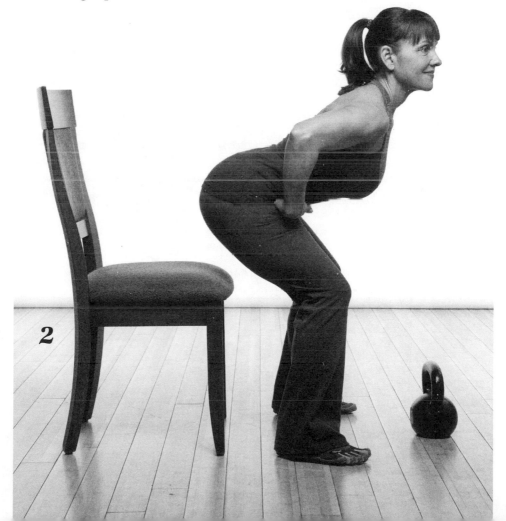

2

The Chair Hike Drill

Now do the Chair Hinge Drill, only this time start with your arms extended out in front of you at hip level (your hands can be placed one on top of the other to help you start to feel the move with two hands). As you hinge back and down, push your arms back and reach for the chair seat with your hands as if you were hiking a ball behind you

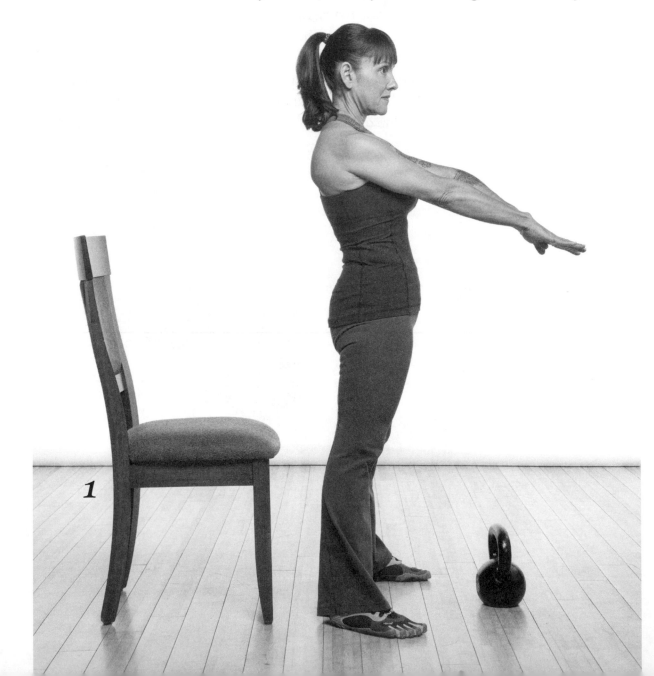

(you don't have to literally "touch" the chair; creating the motion of reaching back is the most important part). You should also feel the outsides of your palms touching the uppermost part of your inner thighs. This connection is what transfers the power of your hips through your arms and hands to the bell. The motion of pushing your arms back and behind you is the start of the kettlebell swing—it begins when you back the bell up.

Once you tap the chair seat with your hands, quickly stand up straight, swinging your hands out in front of you to hip level only. Remember to contract your quads, squeeze your glutes, and exhale sharply as you stand.

Repeat this sequence 5–10 times: hinge back and down, push your arms back, and touch the chair with your hands. Stand up.

You should be feeling the power of the swing about now—just imagine how it's going to feel once you add the kettlebell in!

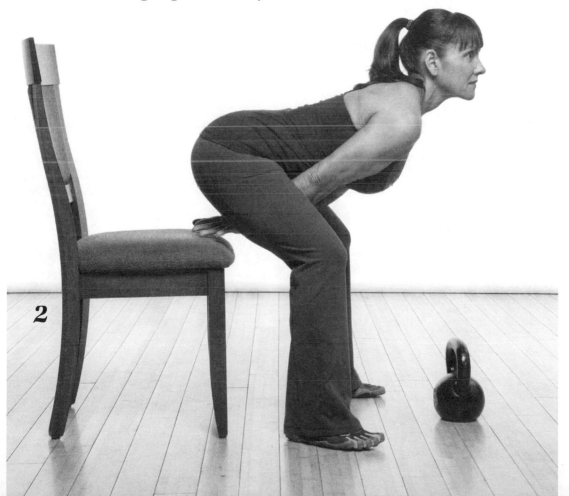

The Single Swing Drill

Return to your position between the kettlebell and your chair. Hinge back and down, reaching out in front of you to touch the handle of the bell. This is your starting and end position for this drill, but you won't be picking up the kettlebell quite yet. The entire sequence will look like this:

Touch the handle of the bell.

Reach back to touch the chair with your hands.

Stand up straight, contracting quads, glutes, and abs, while swinging your arms out in front of you to hip level (not higher).

Hinge back and down again, reaching back to touch the chair with your hands.

Touch the handle of the bell.

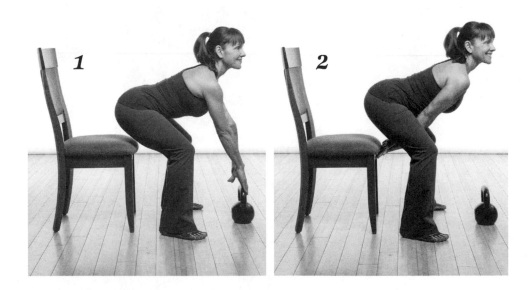

As you stand up, "shake it out"—shake your arms, hands, and legs to release tension you've created while contracting your muscles. This is a good habit to get into after you perform your swings.

If I were teaching you the Single Swing in a class right now, this is how I would guide you through this drill: "Get in position. Now, handle of the bell, touch the chair, stand up swing, touch the chair, handle of the bell. Repeat. Handle of the bell, touch the chair, stand up swing, touch the chair, handle of the bell. Great job!"

This is an excellent sequence to practice over and over again; it will help you start to familiarize your body with the movement of picking up the bell, swinging the bell once, and then putting the bell down. The next exercise will take you through continuous swing movements without "putting the bell down" between each swing.

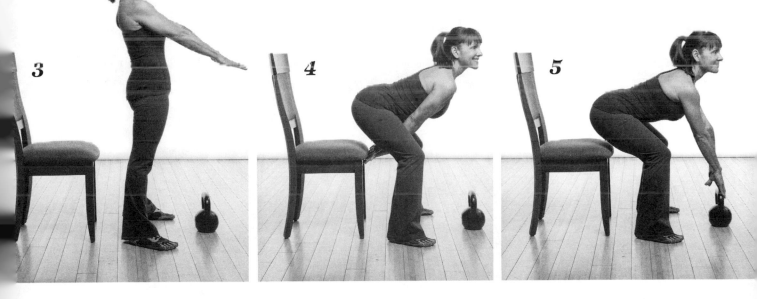

The Air Swing

The swing happens faster than you think. To make sure you're ready for it, I'm going to have you put the Single Swing Drill into more action. This means you'll be performing the sequence consecutively. These are what I call Air Swings, but they're not just for practice, they can be a workout in themselves. Since I've led you through the full description of each part of the movement, I'm going to describe this in simple steps (refer back to the previous steps for comprehensive descriptions).
Try it out:

Touch the handle of the bell.

Reach back and touch the chair.

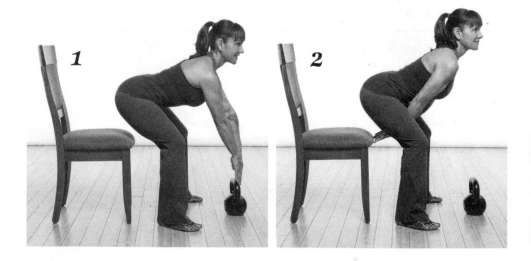

Stand up swing.

Reach back and touch the chair.

Stand up swing.

Reach back and touch the chair.

Stand up swing.

Repeat 7 more times for a total of 10 swings.

After touching the chair one last time, pretend to put the bell down by touching the handle of the bell.

Tired yet?

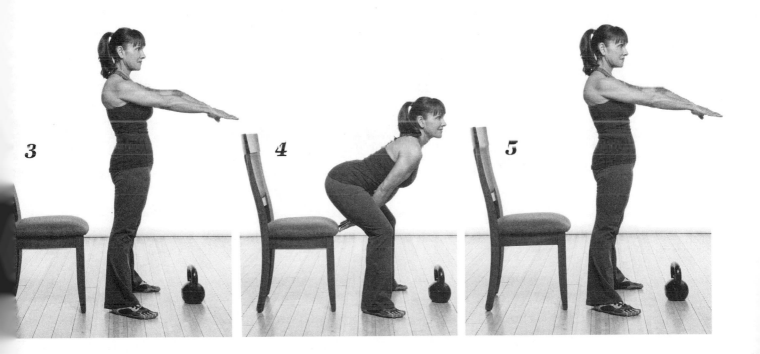

Timed Air Swings

I want to make sure you're starting to get the pace, so now I'm going to have you time your Air Swings. Get a clock with a clearly visible second hand and put it somewhere you can see it. When the second hand gets to the twelve, perform a set of 10 Air Swings. Check your time. How was it? I'm going to guess not quite fast enough. You should be completing 10 Air Swings in fifteen seconds—that's how fast the swing happens! When the second hand gets to the three, you should be finishing your tenth Air Swing. Because pacing is so important with the swing, you must succeed at this pace with Air Swings before moving on to using the bell. I'm trying to make the swing easier for you—once you add the bell in, you'll realize how important pace is.

Have you reached 10 Air Swings in fifteen seconds? You can move on now to the full swing, but for some of you, the Air Swing may have been a workout in itself, and that's okay. If you've broken a sweat and raised your heart rate, congratulations! You've made your first step toward reconnecting with your body. If you don't have a bell yet or you feel that the Air Swings alone were challenging for your body, try this Bell-Free Workout for a week:

The Bell-Free Workout

Complete 3 Single Swings. Rest 10–30 seconds.

Complete 5 Single Swings. Rest 15–45 seconds.

Complete 8 Single Swings. Rest 30–60 seconds.

Complete 10 Single Swings. Rest 30–90 seconds.

Now add in Air Swings:

Complete 8–10 Air Swings. Rest 15–45 seconds.

Repeat entire sequence starting with 3 Single Swings 2–3 more times.

Don't linger too long on just the Air Swings, though—the kettlebell is what's going to create the incredible results (it's what makes this a weight-resistant exercise). So without further delay, let's get to grabbing that bell.

· ·

The Rest That's Right for You

One of the great aspects about your first few workouts is that you decide how much rest you need between sets (you'll notice in the Bell-Free Workout, I've given the rest time a range). This is all based on your level of fitness, taking into consideration your current body weight and/or past or current workout history.

Because you will feel your heart rate increase quickly, it's important to let it come back down so you will be able to perform your next set of swings, but it's equally important that you not take too much rest. A good way to measure is to take the talk test. If you are gasping for air, you haven't given yourself enough rest; if you can hold a conversation, you've had too much rest.

If you have a heart rate monitor, you want it to read around 110 before moving into your next set. Without a monitor, count the number of beats during a six-second interval and multiply by ten to get your heart rate. If you're getting eleven to twelve beats per six seconds, then you're ready to jump back in.

You should be able to perform 8–10 Air Swings without much cardiovascular difficulty, but keep in mind, once you add the weight resistance of the kettlebell, this number of reps will be more difficult and you will, more than likely, need longer rest periods.

· ·

Hike the Bell

Remove the chair so there's a clear space behind you. Now it's just you and the bell, which should be about six inches in front of your feet. Before you do the full swing with a bell, you need to practice one more move, but you are going to use the kettlebell this time.

Stand in front of the bell and get a good grip on the handle with both hands.

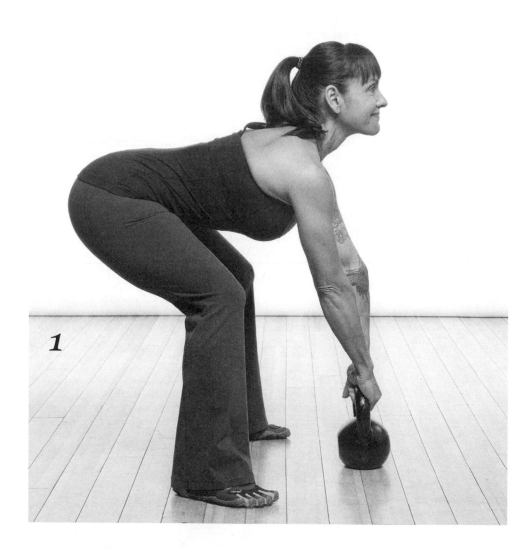

Without standing up, simply hike the kettlebell back and up behind you, re-creating the motion of touching the chair, and then let it swing forward and back to its position on the ground in front of you.

Repeat this 4–5 times.

The important point of this drill is to get used to the weight of the bell and to focus on creating the angle of the movement—you are hiking it back and up at the same time. Remember, like a kid on a swing, you have to back up first. The force you create by pushing the bell back and up is what creates the momentum for the kettlebell to float out and swing in front of your body. Don't be afraid if you hit your butt with the bell; that's actually good at this point.

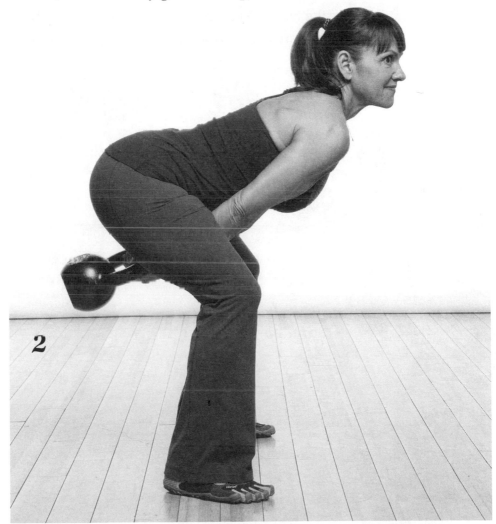

2

The Swing

Are you ready to swing? I know I am! You've already done Air Swings, so you've familiarized your body with the movement, and you've hiked the weight back, so you know what it feels like to have the kettlebell weight in your hands—now it's time to put it all together. Remember, you are going to perform the same movement as the Air Swing, only with a bell in your hands—don't overthink it. The swing is a very natural movement, and once you feel it done right, you won't ever forget it—just like riding a bike.

Just like with the last drill, I want you to put the bell about six inches in front of you on the ground. Here's the complete swing, broken down into steps.

Hike back and up

1

Stand up swing, bringing your extended arms to about hip height

2

Obviously you can't read the steps as you're swinging so read through them, then jump right up to do your swings, and don't forget—it's supposed to be fun!

End by bending your knees, letting the bell swing behind you and then land out in front as you softly place it back on the ground.

That's the swing! It might be hard to believe, but that is the move that helped me lose nearly 120 pounds and transform my body.

You can continue to practice with the swing and see how it feels, but as soon as you're ready, I recommend getting started with the workouts beginning on page 121. Now that you understand the basics of the swing, I'm going to use the rest of this chapter to give you some modifications, refinements, and form fixes.

Hinge back and down while reaching and pushing the bell behind you

3

Stand up swing

Repeat 8–10 times

4

A Simple Modification: Towel Swings

If you are having difficulty grabbing the bell with two hands in front of your body because of your size, then you can practice what are known as Towel Swings. You will practice all of the beginning drills without the bell: hinging; reaching back toward the seat of a chair with your arms; standing up and contracting your glutes, quads, and abs; and so on. You will practice Air Swings and Timed Air Swings. Only when it comes time to practice with the bell, will you do anything differently. Just use a towel to extend your reach to the handle. All this does is make it easier for you to use your hips. The extended reach created by the towel will make your hinging movement shallower, but this will create just as good of a workout for you, if not better. The extension makes it difficult to use your arms and forces you to use your hips.

To perform a Towel Swing, thread a towel through the handle of the bell and grip both ends of the towel as close to the handle as possible.

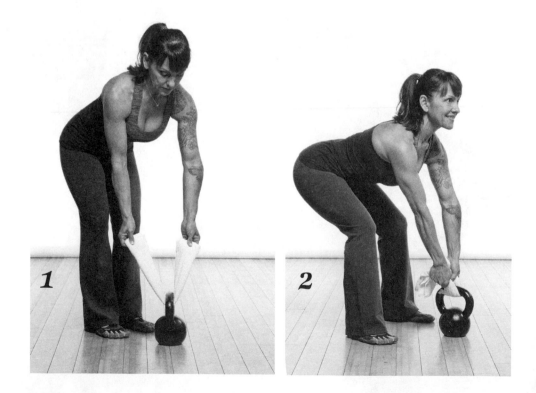

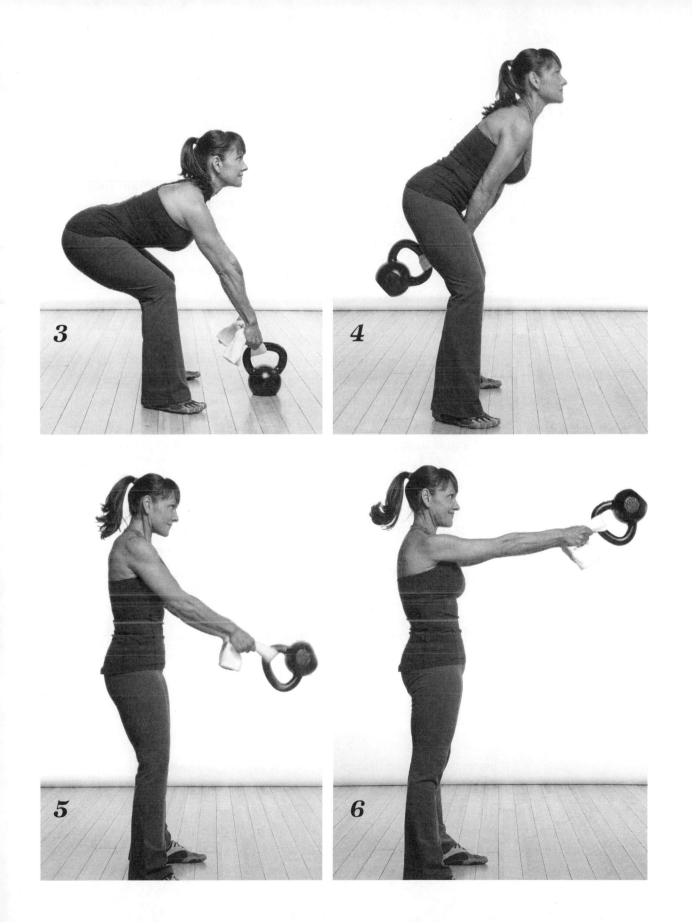

Breathing

How you breathe during a kettlebell swing is very important for your back health and safety. Proper breathing will also allow for increased performance. The technical term for breathing correctly is diaphragmatic breathing, but for the sake of simplicity we'll call it belly breathing. Belly breathing is not only the right way to breathe while doing your kettlebell workouts; it's the best way to breathe in everyday life.

The diaphragm is a large, umbrella shaped muscle right under your rib cage. Most people are chest breathers, meaning their breathing occurs up in the chest and never dips down into the diaphragm. When you keep breathing in your chest, you rob yourself of two-thirds of the oxygen you could be getting. Oxygen does more than just keep us alive—it energizes our cells and tissues, and fuels our muscles, which is especially important during a workout.

If you pay attention to your own breathing motion, you'll probably notice the movement stays in the chest as the top of the shoulders (trapezius muscle, also known as traps) literally lift the ribs off the lungs to let them take in air. This is very inefficient, and it creates tight traps and neck, causes headaches, and diminishes energy.

To breathe correctly, your belly should actually move out when you inhale and in when you exhale. Think of how little kids breathe when they are out of breath, and you will know what belly breathing looks like. Their little tummies go in and out like a bellows, while their shoulders hardly move.

To learn to belly breathe, place your hand on your stomach and as you inhale, make your belly button move forward. As you exhale try to pull your belly button toward your spine—you should feel the movement in your belly; if you don't, you are breathing from your chest. Most people, especially women, find this quite difficult at first, as so many are taught to never let their stomachs out. This can lead to all kinds of problems, such as lower back pain, tight trapezius muscles, headaches, neck aches, and a general inability to stabilize the core.

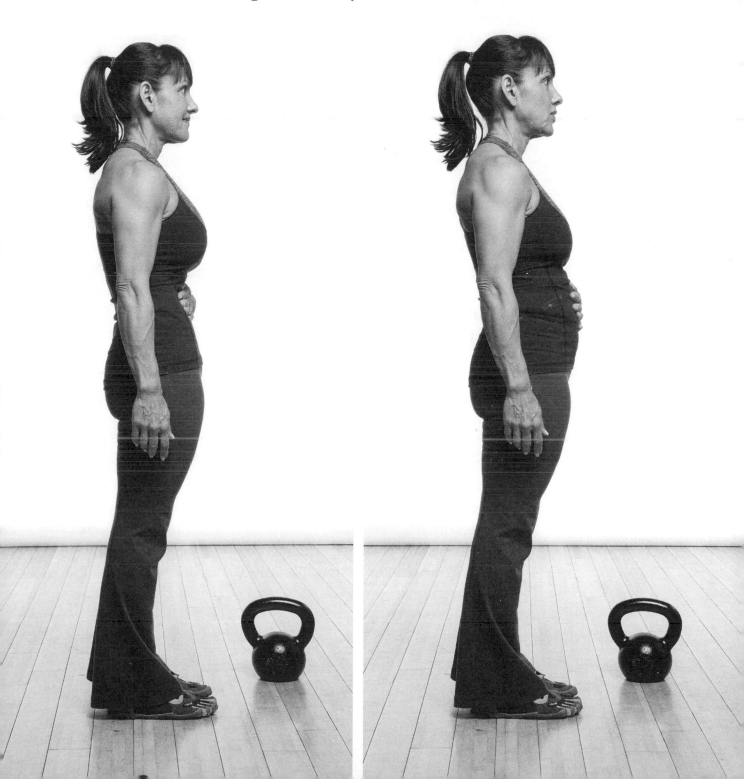

So go ahead—give yourself permission to stick your stomach out. The good news is that letting your stomach out on the inhalation will work your muscles in a way that will tighten your waistline. These muscles (the transversus abdominus) are like a muscular corset that will tighten your waist on every breath.

Here's a quick tip to make belly breathing easier: inhale through your nose. If you do this, it is much easier to breathe into the belly than if you try to do so through your mouth. Place your hand on your stomach, and try this exercise: breathe in through your nose as you make the belly button move forward. Then, exhale through the mouth as you pull the navel in.

During your kettlebell swings, inhale through the nose as the bell swings behind you, and exhale through the mouth on the upswing. Drawing your belly in and exhaling at the top of the swing is good, but bracing your abs is even better. To do this, imagine that someone is trying to punch you in the stomach. The best way to protect yourself from this punch is to "tighten up" your abs—this is how you should brace your abdominal muscles at the top of the swing. As you are bracing your abs, you should be letting out a short, sharp exhale (you can either hiss some air out or count your rep number). Inhale through the nose for the next rep, and repeat. Don't worry—this will become perfectly natural in a very short time.

If the concept of bracing your abs seems tough for you to get, you can practice by doing something that may sound a bit silly, but it's the easiest way to understand the feeling. So here it goes—I want you to punch yourself in the stomach. Do it gently at first, and then progressively hit a bit harder as you learn to tighten your entire core just before your fist makes contact. Believe me, this is the easiest and quickest way to learn how to contract your muscles (and it's definitely smarter than having someone else punch you!).

One of the best parts of kettlebell swing training is all the development you get in areas you don't think are being worked by the swing. Using the belly breathing technique makes every move more efficient and will ensure your abs get an amazing workout on each rep of every swing. Just think: you'll never have to do a single crunch again.

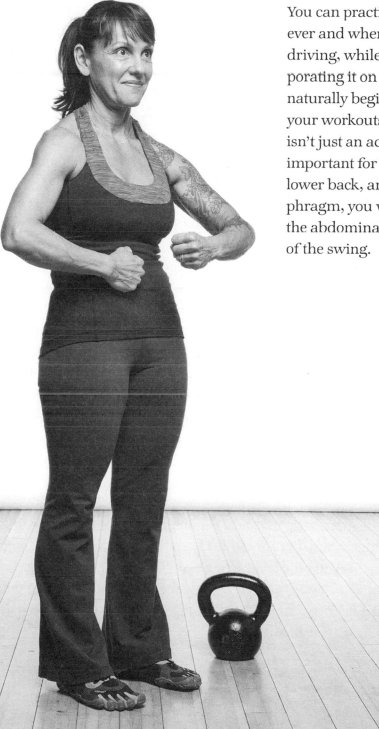

You can practice belly breathing whenever and wherever—in your office, while driving, while watching TV. Start incorporating it on a regular basis so you naturally begin to breathe this way in your workouts. This breathing technique isn't just an accessory to the swing; it's important for the protection of your lower back, and by engaging the diaphragm, you will automatically activate the abdominal muscles at the bottom of the swing.

Contraction

At the top of every swing, you want to make sure to tighten up your thighs, glutes, and abs; to grip the floor with your feet; and to keep your shoulders pulled into the sockets. When you incorporate each of these elements, you accomplish several things that will be important to creating the results you want (and to keeping your workouts safe):

- You ensure lower-body stability and make sure the bell doesn't pull you out of position.

- You protect your knees, back, and shoulders by creating a muscular contraction to stabilize the joints.

- You create tone and strength in all of these areas.

  If any of these areas are loose, you create a power leakage (a term often used in the RKC). Since the body is a linked and interconnected system, any leakage in one area will reduce total body strength and prevent you from developing a fully beneficial momentum. More importantly, power leakages can also create opportunities for injury—a body part that's not fully contracted is one with which you can easily lose connection.

  As you perform the swing, think about your hips and glutes as the engines of the movement. The arms and shoulders, on the other hand, are just tethered to the bell and do not raise the weight, but they still must be contracted and connected to the bell at all times.

  One of the most basic mistakes beginners make is quickly letting go of the glute contraction. You must keep the buns tight for as long as possible, releasing the contraction right before the bell swings between your legs. Otherwise the weight of the bell will really want to pull you forward. Squeeze your glutes at the top of the swing, and keep them tight for as long as possible.

To practice this, a good exercise is one similar to a bridge pose in yoga. Lie on the ground on your back and lift your hips up toward the ceiling by tightening your glute muscles. Hold this position, squeezing your glutes and keeping your hips lifted. Now stand up and perform 10 swings recreating the feeling of that hip extension every time you stand up with the bell.

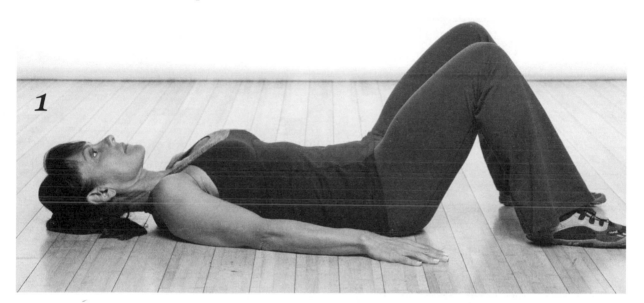

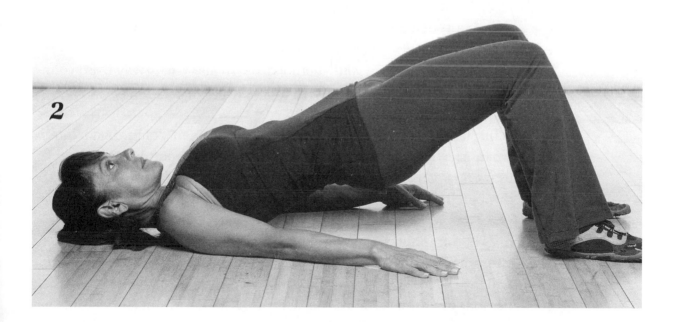

Tightening the front of the thighs at the top of the swing will allow you to safely straighten the legs fully. If you don't tighten the thighs, the leg can still straighten, but it won't have the muscular contraction to keep it safe. You want to straighten the leg, not hyperextend it, so be sure to tighten your thighs. This will also give your thighs fantastic muscle tone and strength without ever doing squats.

If you have knee issues and can't squat, you can still swing safely and easily, and strengthen the knees and legs at the same time. Swings are perhaps the most knee-friendly, full-body exercise a person can do at any age.

Contracting the shoulder into the socket is vital for shoulder health and a powerful swing. When you come out of the bottom position, you will find your shoulder is already perfectly where it should be. The only reason it might come forward is if you let your arms power the ascent instead of the hips. Keep the shoulders tightly in their sockets as you let your hips and glutes propel the bell upward. Remember, you are swinging the bell, not lifting it.

An easy way to feel if your shoulders are following proper form is to feel what it's like when they are not. Extend your arms out in front of you about shoulder height, and lift your shoulders up toward your ears (out of the socket), now pull them down and back away from your ears (in the socket). Pulling your shoulders down and back away from your ears automatically keeps your shoulder packed.

While it's important to keep all of this in mind, I don't want you to think too much while you're swinging. When it comes to contraction, the important point is to stay connected to your body and muscles as you go through the swing. You accomplish this by simply paying attention. This process is about transforming your body, but it all starts by opening the lines of communication. With each swing, think about the contractions of your muscles as an act of squeezing the weight off of you—I'm sure that will help you feel connected to the movements! No matter what, remember that you want to control the kettlebell; you don't want it to control you.

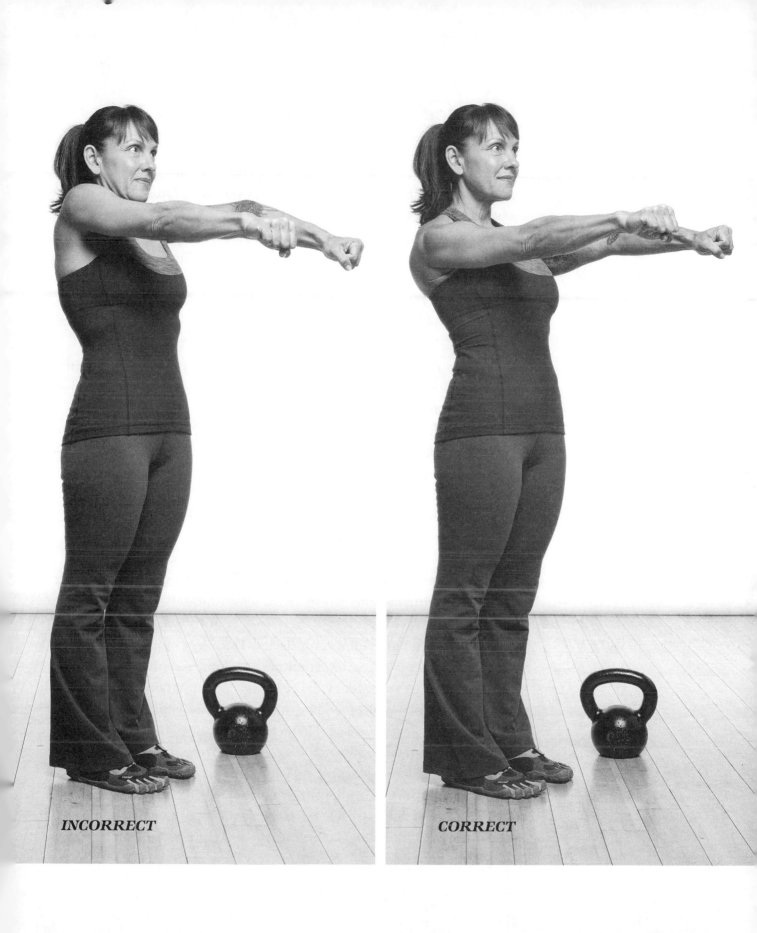

INCORRECT

CORRECT

The Difference Between Soreness and Pain

The day after your first kettlebell workout, you will probably experience soreness in your inner thighs like you've never felt before. Don't worry—it's normal and it's unavoidable. When you swing the weight between your legs, it stretches those muscles in a way that they're not stretched by regular activities, even other exercise activities. The good news is that once you get through that break-in period, you won't get very sore again anywhere on your body. Think of this initial soreness as a rite of passage into the Kettlebell Swing Club.

The workload in a kettlebell swing is so evenly distributed throughout your entire body that no single area gets isolated or overloaded, which is why, other than in your inner thighs, you don't feel much soreness after your first workout. The even distribution is also why your perception of your efforts during your workout is lower than in traditional methods—your whole body is helping, so it doesn't seem like any one part of you is doing all the work. Since everything is being put to work during the swing, you can burn an outrageous number of calories and change your body rapidly with super short workouts.

However, it is still common to feel some soreness when you are beginning or increasing the intensity of an exercise routine. It is important that you not confuse the effort of exercising your muscles, heart, and lungs hard with pain in joints or muscles. They are completely different. Taking your body to a new level of fitness and into a reinvented existence altogether requires that you push past old limitations, which is rarely comfortable. While it will be uncomfortable—your body might feel a bit tired and your muscles tender for a day or two—this is a different sensation than what you would experience from injury-related pain, which is sharp and long-lasting. As you begin to reconnect with your body, you'll become more adept at gauging the difference. When it comes to injuries, there are a few red flags you should watch out for—areas where you should not be feeling much soreness, if any at all.

Warning Signs and Quick Fixes

As you perform more swings, I want you to be able to self-correct when you feel something is off with the movement. Here are some warning signs you might encounter if your form isn't quite right, and some simple adjustments to fix it.

Warning: Shoulder Pain

When I say shoulder pain, I'm including the trapezius muscles, which people often incorrectly identify as their shoulder. Your traps are directly to the side of the neck, while the shoulders are the muscles at the end of your collarbones. Either way, neither of these parts of your body should hurt from swinging a kettlebell. If you're experiencing pain in your shoulders or traps, you're using your arms instead of your hips to pull the weight out of the bottom position.

Quick Fix: Try a shallow swing just below hip level, make sure to keep your elbows straight as you go through your repetitions, and use your hips to create the movement of the swing, not your arms. When the bell goes up, your shoulders come down.

Warning: Lower Back Pain

Your lower back should not hurt from swinging a kettlebell. If it does, check to make sure you're keeping a straight spine (see the straight spine section on page 86). If you're not maintaining the four natural curves of the spine, you are letting the lower back round, which is the main cause of any lower back pain.

Quick Fix: Maintain a slight arch, not a rounding, in the lower back throughout the entire movement and use the hips to create the swing.

Ensuring your hamstrings are flexible and mobile will help as well, as tight hamstrings will pull on the pelvis and make it harder to maintain a solid back arch. To stretch out your hamstrings, try this (you can use a belt if you don't have a strap):

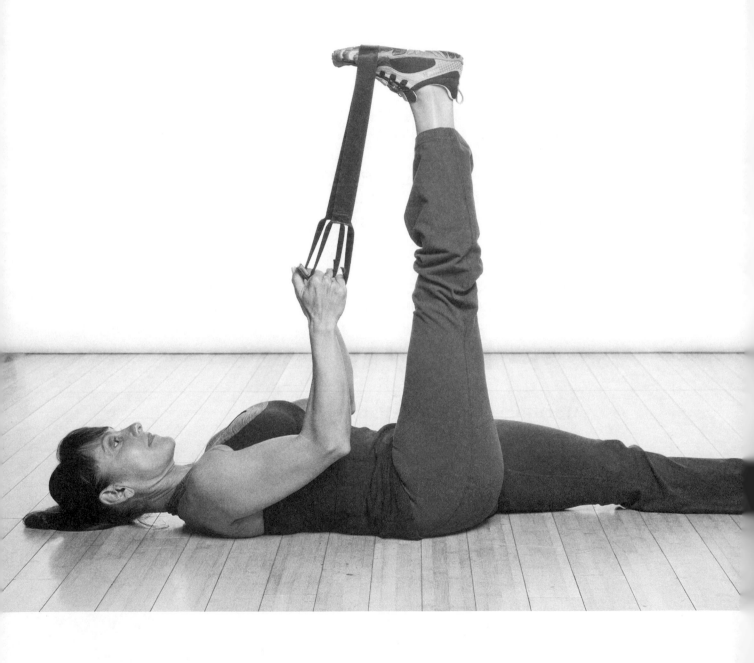

Warning: Knee Pain

The knees should always track the toes. This means that whatever direction your toes are pointed when you're swinging is the direction your knees should be pointing as well. Your knees and feet should be pointed straight ahead, or at the most at twenty degrees outward.

Quick Fix: Don't let your knees cave in, and make sure to keep your feet flat on the floor the entire time—don't let yourself go up on your toes or let the big toes come off the ground. To make sure you are hinging and not squatting, pay attention to where the swing breaks—it should happen at the hips, and not at the knees. Stretching out your quads can also help make sure your legs are ready for the swing. Try this stretch:

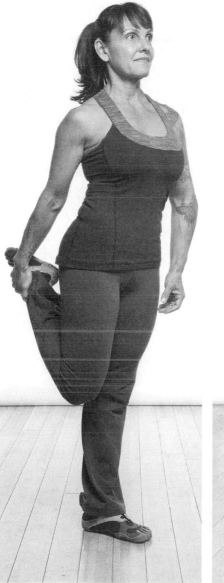

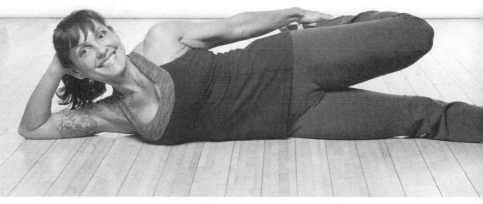

The Kettlebell Triangle

The Chair Hinge and Chair Hike Drills should have taught you the precise path your hands should follow during the swing. When you do the swing correctly, this means your hands should pass right below your groin area, and I mean right below. When you have a moving kettlebell in your hands, you now have a combined center of gravity between you and the bell. Your center is your belly button. The bell's center, because of the handle, is somewhere near the top of the ball of iron. The combined center, the one between you and the bell, is in the triangle created by your groin area and your pubic bone—what I call the kettlebell triangle. If you feel like you are being pulled forward and

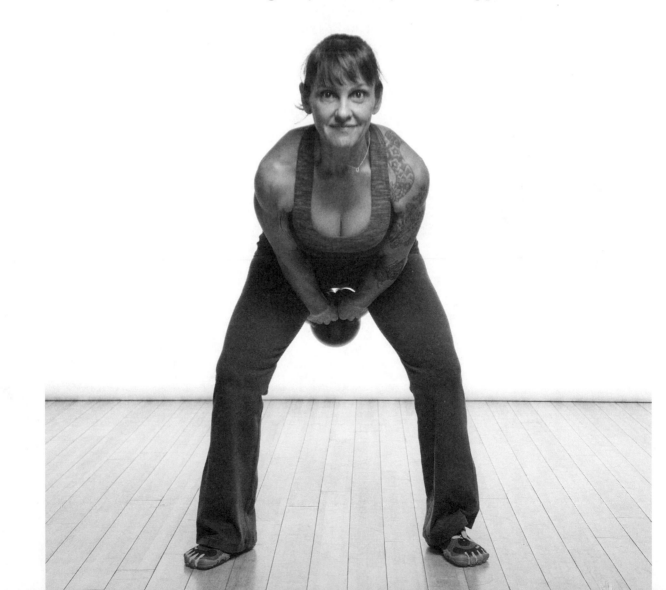

down by the bell, then you have simply strayed too far away from your center of gravity, or the kettlebell triangle.

When you swing the kettlebell, you should be re-creating the motion of reaching back and up to touch the chair; if you follow this arc, you will ensure your hands stay within the triangle. It is most common to be pulled away from the triangle when you try swinging the bell with one hand, but it can happen in the Two-Hand Swing as well. This is an example of when it would be okay to use a mirror to help you correct this mistake—stand in front of one and practice to make sure you're keeping the bell at the top part of the triangle. Remember to only use the mirror to make form corrections and refinements—once you've got the motion and positioning down, move the mirror out of the way so you can focus completely on your body instead of on a reflection.

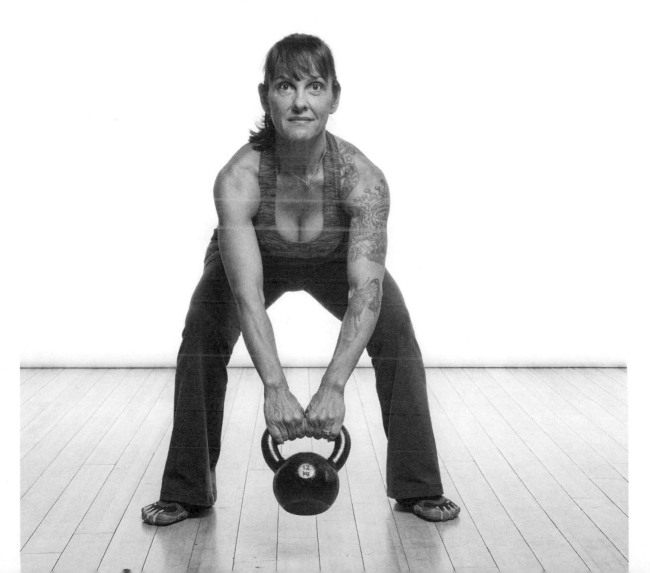

A Final Tip

Before you start the workouts, I want you to remind you to really focus on your body and how the swing feels. Ever since I started teaching others how to swing, I've noticed that the biggest mistake people make is overthinking and not feeling the movement of the swing. I've certainly given you plenty to think about in this chapter, but I don't want you to get lost in your head or to feel overwhelmed by the details. When you try the swing, I think you'll be surprised to discover how easy it is; let the details refine as you improve your skills, but don't be afraid to lift your eyes off the page and get comfortable with the swing through repetitions.

9

The Swing Workouts

Now that you have been a student of the swing and have put in your time in rehearsal, it's time to step onto the big stage of the workouts—this is where you'll really ramp up the caloric burn and body transformation. As I guide you through the workouts in this next phase, Practice, I want you to think of them as recipes for success.

In each of the different types of workouts I'm going to offer here, I'll give you a brief description of the workout structure, then the specifics relating to reps, sets, and rest time—these figures are the measurements I've worked with over the years and have refined to the point where they create the perfect workout. Initially, I modified the workouts with the purpose of progressively challenging my body, but once I started teaching classes and instructing others, I really focused also on making the workouts fun—that is, I developed ways for people to perform extraordinary workloads in a very short amount of time. The fun comes through just a bit of deception—you won't even realize how much you're getting done in just thirty minutes or less (of course, until you see the results in the mirror). As you become more familiar with the workouts, I want you to think of them like measurements for a favorite recipe—they can be manipulated and customized to better suit your taste or fitness level.

I use what's known as interval training to create most of my workouts for *The Swing!* Interval training is a method that alternates levels of output, most often going from bursts of intense effort to a resting or low-intensity interval. This type of training is incredibly effective at improving your body strength and increasing your cardiovascular endurance.

The first goal of timed interval swing training is what I call equal work to equal rest. This means if you swing for thirty seconds, then you rest for thirty seconds. The number of reps you do is not as important as establishing the rest it takes you to recover and swing more reps. The stronger you get and the more your cardiovascular endurance improves, the shorter amount of rest you will require. Equal work to equal rest is the baseline level of cardio endurance required to move from the Practice phase to the Training phase. It may take weeks if not months to establish this ratio of work to rest, but the good news is that your progress is so individual that you need not compare your ability to anyone else's—it's based solely on your last workout. I'm going to teach you how to work your way up to equal work to equal rest with something I call On the Minute training—this is a simple way to use a set time frame to organize your workouts.

The Practice Phase: Workouts #1–5

In this phase, I'm going to have you perform your workouts on the minute, which means that every set will start at the beginning of every minute, or when the second hand reaches the twelve on a clock. You will start one set of swings at the top of each minute, regardless of how many reps you've completed or how much rest you've gotten. On the Minute (OTM) training is an uncomplicated way of structuring your workouts because you don't have to time your reps or your rest period; you only have to time the intervals.

We will be using one-minute intervals. Remember, within each one-minute interval, you incorporate work and rest. The only move we will be using in the first five workouts is the Two-Hand Swing. At any point, though, you can opt for Air Swings if you can't continue to swing the kettlebell—the important part is to keep swinging.

On the Minute Workout #1

Perform 10 swing reps for 5 sets OTM. Remember, this means that you will complete 5 sets with a clock with a second hand nearby—each time you've completed 10 Two-Hand Swings, look up at the clock and see how much time is left to "finish the minute." It should be around forty-five seconds, give or take five seconds; this will all depend on your ability to set the pace of 10 reps per fifteen seconds.

After your first 5 sets, it's time to evaluate. Did you get too much rest or not enough rest? If you felt it was too much rest, you can move right on to OTM Workout #2. If you did not get enough rest, decrease your number of reps to 8 and repeat 5 more sets on the minute. Now reevaluate. If you feel like you got too much rest, increase your reps back up to 10. If you feel like you didn't get enough rest, add an extra minute rest at this time (giving you a rest time of one minute and forty-five seconds) and then decrease to 5 or 6 reps. If you felt it was just right, continue on with 8–10 reps and repeat 5 more sets. It is not uncommon to have to decrease the rep count in the first couple of workouts, but your cardio fitness will improve quickly with every consistent workout.

For OTM Workouts #1–5, you might find it helpful to keep track of the number of sets you've completed and what kind of work-to-rest ratio you are keeping. A work-to-rest ratio is simply the amount of time you spent doing work, or swinging, and the amount time you spent resting.

It doesn't have to be exact—just keep an eye on the average for each group of 5 sets of 10 reps. Since you practiced pacing your Air Swings, you should average around fifteen seconds for every set of 10 swings, followed by forty-five seconds of rest. This is a 1:3 work-to-rest ratio.

I'm going to be using shorthand when giving you your workout instructions, as it will be much easier for you when you get to the more advanced workouts. You will find a complete key on page 139, but this is the only one you will need to know until Workout #6 (it's pretty obvious):

2-hd sw = two-hand swings

The Swing!	**OTM WORKOUT #1**		
Swings	**Sets**	**Sets Completed**	**Work/Rest**
10 2-hd sw	5		
8–10 2-hd sw	5		
5–10 2-hd sw	5		
Total Workout Time: 15 minutes			
Notes:			

On the Minute Workout #2

This workout is 15 sets. You will start with 10 reps for the first 5 sets, then you add 1 rep each set until you reach 15 reps. This is the goal, but it's important to gauge how you feel—did you reach your limit at 12 or 14? Once you find the number of reps that creates the ideal workout for you, repeat that number until you've completed 15 sets total.

The Swing!	OTM WORKOUT #2		
Swings	**Sets**	**Sets Completed**	**Work/Rest**
10 2-hd sw	5		
_____ 2-hd sw	1		
_____ 2-hd sw	1		
_____ 2-hd sw	1		
_____ 2-hd sw	1		
_____ 2-hd sw	1		
_____ 2-hd sw	5		
Total Workout Time: 15 minutes			
Notes:			

On the Minute Workout #3

This workout is 20 sets. You will start with 10 reps, increasing 1 swing per set until you reach 20 reps. Once you find the number of reps that creates the right challenge for you, repeat that number until you've completed 20 sets total.

The Swing!	OTM WORKOUT #3		
Swings	**Sets**	**Sets Completed**	**Work/Rest**
10 2-hd sw	5		
____ 2-hd sw	1		
____ 2-hd sw	1		
____ 2-hd sw	1		
____ 2-hd sw	1		
____ 2-hd sw	1		
____ 2-hd sw	1		
____ 2-hd sw	1		
____ 2-hd sw	1		
____ 2-hd sw	1		
____ 2-hd sw	1		
____ 2-hd sw	5		
Total Workout Time: 20 minutes			
Notes:			

Continue with Workout #3 (again beginning with 1 set of 10, increasing 1 rep at a time) until you've reached the fitness level where you can complete 20 reps within thirty seconds, which will mean you're getting thirty seconds of work to thirty seconds of rest. Once you've reached that point, let me wish you congratulations because you have reached equal work to equal rest! This is a great accomplishment in itself because it represents great progress in your cardio endurance. Don't celebrate for too long, though—if you want to achieve your best body, you've got to continue pushing progress by upping the challenge. With that, let's move on to Workout #4.

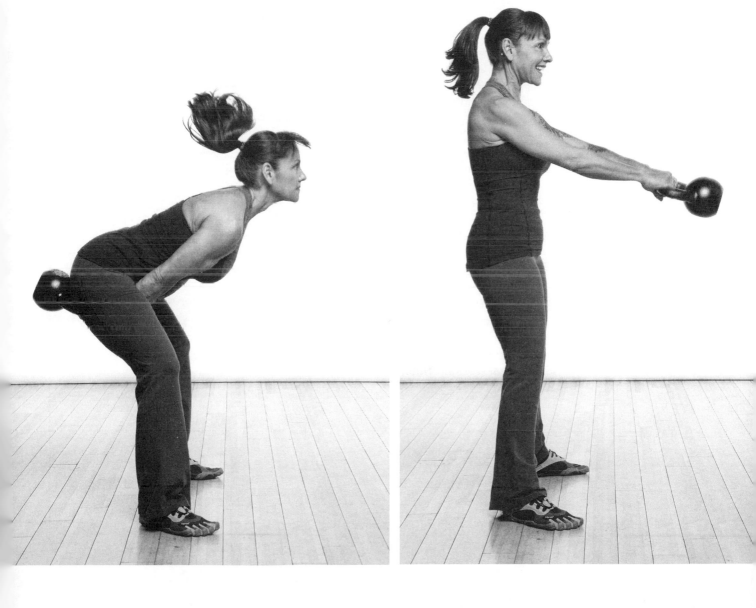

On the Minute Workout #4

We're going to increase the challenge here by starting with 12 reps, and then we'll increase each set at first by 1 rep, then by 2, and we will end with 10–15 sets of 20 reps.

The Swing!	**OTM WORKOUT #4**		
Swings	**Sets**	**Sets Completed**	**Work/Rest**
12 2-hd sw	1		
____ 2-hd sw	1		
____ 2-hd sw	1		
____ 2-hd sw	1		
____ 2-hd sw	1		
____ 2-hd sw	1		
____ 2-hd sw	1		
____ 2-hd sw	1		
____ 2-hd sw	1		
____ 2-hd sw	1		
20 2-hd sw	10–15		
Total Workout Time: 20–25 minutes			
Notes:			

On the Minute Workout #5

This is your last OTM workout. Great job so far—you're probably noticing amazing changes in your body, including increased cardio endurance, significant weight loss, and impressive muscle shape and tone. How quickly the muscle tone reveals itself will depend on how much weight you have to lose—remember, as your weight drops, so does your body fat, and getting that out of the way will allow your muscle tone to really show off.

With this final OTM workout, you'll start with 12 reps and increase each following set by 2 reps until you reach 20 reps. Then you will complete 10–20 sets of 20 reps, and finish with 20 reps or any of the previous rep counts (the most you can do) for 10 more sets. With this last group of sets, just do your best each set. If you find you're not getting enough rest, drop back down to 12 reps and work your way up again. The most important point is to finish with 10 sets, regardless of the rep count.

The Swing! OTM WORKOUT #5			
Swings	**Sets**	**Sets Completed**	**Work/Rest**
12 2-hd sw	1		
____ 2-hd sw	1		
____ 2-hd sw	1		
____ 2-hd sw	1		
____ 2-hd sw	1		
20 2-hd sw	10–20		
____ 2-hd sw	10		
Total Workout Time: 25–30 minutes			
Notes:			

Just Keep Swinging

The important part to remember for all these workouts is that you can always work at your own pace. In other words, if you need more rest, then take it. All swing workouts can be customized to your level of fitness. Don't worry that you are not doing enough. If you are doing your swing workout consistently—that's the key—you will improve quickly, and you may even experience your cardio endurance has doubled from one workout to the next. The results and the physical progress will happen quickly.

The other benefit of your kettlebell swing training is that it doesn't set you up to get into the bad habit of comparing yourself to others. Everyone has a unique starting point. Even if you have the same amount of weight to lose as someone else, your cardiovascular fitness could be greater or lesser than that person's. I often use the analogy of drinking alcohol. If you don't drink alcohol often, then you may feel tipsy after one glass. Whereas someone who drinks alcohol on a regular basis probably needs three or more glasses before he feels the effects. Neither one is better—they're both getting tipsy. I may be able to swing for minutes at a time, but your 10 swings are doing you every bit of good as my minutes of swings—it's all relative.

You may be able to perform 20 swing reps easily now, but how many sets of 20 can you complete with equal rest before tiring out? As I mentioned, the rep count is not as important as how many sets of reps you can complete using the equal-work-to-equal-rest ratio. The goal is to progressively increase the number of consecutive intervals you can do.

Stop! Read This Before You Move On

At this point, you have established two important skills: 1) You can complete 10 reps per fifteen seconds, or 20 reps per thirty seconds, and 2) you can complete your reps with equal work to equal rest, which translates to being able to work 10 reps and rest into a thirty-second interval, or 20 reps and rest into a one-minute interval. To extend a bit further, this means you should be able to complete 5 sets of 10 Two-Hand Swing reps in two-and-a-half minutes (5 sets × 30 seconds each = 2.5 minutes total), or 5 sets of 20 Two-Hand Swing reps in five minutes (5 sets × one-minute each = five minutes).

All the workouts moving forward will assume that you've achieved this level of skill with your kettlebell workouts. If you haven't gotten to this point yet, keep going with Workouts #1–5, and you will get here— I promise!

The Train Phase: Workouts #6–13

In my opinion, the Two-Hand Swing is the Holy Grail. In terms of difficulty, it is the hardest to train, but it's the simplest to learn. Since both arms are tethered to the bell and involved at all times, there is no rest, but the strength and balance you get from using two hands allows you to safely swing heavier weights. At this point, you could opt to continue to train with just the Two-Hand Swing by working your way up to 40 consecutive reps, 1–2 swings at a time. You could also increase the weight of the bell for some or all of your sets. However, there are convincing reasons to incorporate moves like the One-Hand Swing.

The One-Hand Swing can give at least one side of your body a bit of rest while you keep working with the other. With the Two-Hand Swing your forearms and grip never get a break, which can make it difficult to swing past 20–40 continuous reps. Adding in the One-Hand Swing also gives you variety and helps keep your workouts interesting as your skill with the swing progresses.

In this next phase, Train, you'll discover Workouts #6–13, which will incorporate variations of the One-Hand Swing and plenty of different combinations. First things first though—let's get you comfortable swinging with one arm. Ready to learn it? Let's get to it.

One-Hand Swing

The One-Hand Swing is an asymmetrical movement that forces the body to use 50 percent more muscle. On the flip side of this, the bell will feel about fifty percent heavier because the balance of the weight is off center (see page 73 for weight selection for the One-Hand Swing). This is why it's especially important to get the movement before putting the bell into motion.

To help you establish good from and familiarity with the motion, I want you to revisit the Single Swing Drill (see page 94), but this time I want you to do it with one hand at a time. Don't worry about your free hand or arm for now; I'll instruct you on what to do with it once you've got the concept of the One-Hand Swing down. With the kettlebell out in front of you, hinge back and down and start with your right hand touching the handle (don't pick it up). Push your right arm back and up as if you were going to touch the seat of a chair; now stand up swing, hinge, reach back, pretend to touch the chair, and stand up swing. Switch and perform this drill with your left hand and left arm. Now you're ready to pick up the bell.

Start with your feet hip distance apart with the bell about six inches out in front of you. Hinge down and back and place one hand firmly on the handle of the bell. You will naturally gravitate toward your dominant side—this is fine, but you're going to have to do both sides eventually!

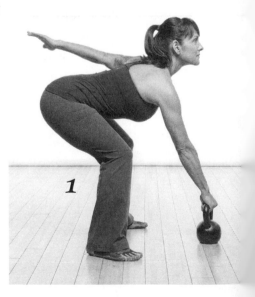

1

Just like with the Single Swing Drill, hike the bell back and up as if you were trying to touch the chair seat behind you.

Stand up swing, contracting your quads and glutes, and sharply exhale at the top.

Push the bell back behind you.

Stand up swing.

Repeat for a total of 5 swings, and then with control, place the bell down in front of you where you began.

Switch hands while the bell is on the ground in front of you. Perform 5 swings with the opposite arm.

Practice One-Hand Swings only a couple of more times on each side, placing the bell down between sets of 5 reps. Now move on to the next drill.

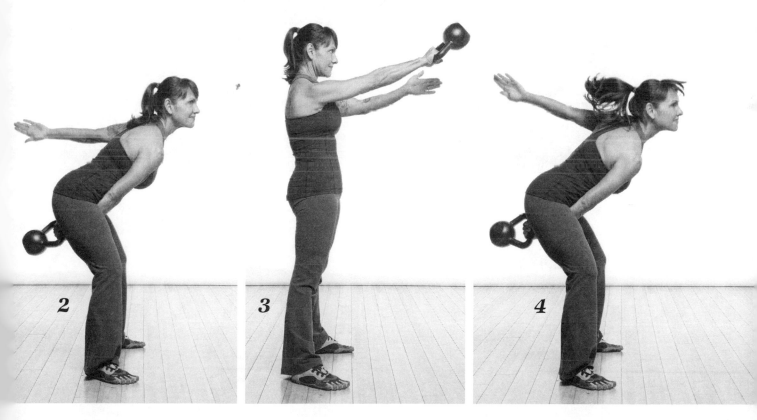

Touch the Handle Drill

It's time to put the free hand and arm to work. This next drill will not only teach you what to do with your free hand and arm, but it will also set you up to switch hands in midair. Sound like fun? It is! Just like when we used the Timed Air Swings to get you ready for the speed of the swing, the Touch the Handle Drill will get you used to the timing of the hand-to-hand switch. The kettlebell is actually floating at only one brief point of the swing, and that's at the very top of each rep. Once you hit that point, you'll need to be ready to transfer hands, which isn't difficult but does require some practice and planning.

Place the bell about six inches out in front of you. With your feet hip distance apart, hinge down and back and place one hand firmly on the handle of the bell. Hike the bell back and up as if you were trying to touch the chair seat behind you.

Stand up swing, and this time touch the handle of the bell with your free hand as the bell swings forward out in front of you.

Push the bell back behind you, and swing your free arm back much like a speed skater does.

Stand up swing; touch the handle with your free hand.

Repeat for 5–10 swings, touching the handle with your free hand each time. Then, with control, place the bell down in front of you.

Switch arms and repeat.

Coach Yourself: You can coach yourself through this drill by repeating the steps out loud. It should sound like this: "Swing touch one, swing touch two, swing touch three, swing touch four, swing touch five, put the bell down." Switch the bell to your other arm, and then repeat.

Practice this way for a few more sets before attempting to switch hands midair. You should start to feel the movement and how important it is to keep your free arm swinging and in sync with your weighted arm. You can count this practice as a workout itself, or you can add on some of your previous Two-Hand Swings for 10–15 sets of 10–20 reps, equal work to rest.

The Touch the Handle Drill is a perfect way to practice the timing of the transfer, but it also has additional benefits. By getting into the habit of swinging your free arm back and forth, you're using up to 35 percent more power (i.e., burning more calories and building more strength). It's also part of the natural gait cycle, like running or walking, and it incorporates the normal thoracic spinal rotation. Not to mention the fact that it feels amazing and athletic, and it creates beautiful artistry in motion. I've gotten into the habit of always swinging my free arm for all these reasons—it feels incredibly natural and powerful.

Hand-to-Hand Switch

Now you're going to learn how to transfer the bell in midair. For obvious reasons, do not practice actually transferring hands in front of a mirror. Keep in mind that the transfer happens on the way up, not on the way down.

Get into position for your one-arm swings. Complete 4 reps with one arm, touching the handle with your free arm each time.

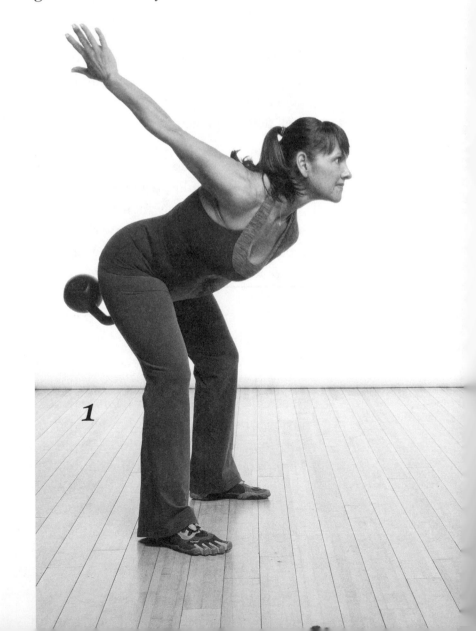

1

On the fifth rep, as your free hand comes toward the handle, pass it over the top of the weighted hand, and then release the weighted hand as you allow the bell to continue its upward path into the top hand. When the bell starts its descent, it should already be in your other hand.

Complete 4 more reps with this opposite arm, switching back on five. Then, with control, place the bell down in front of you.

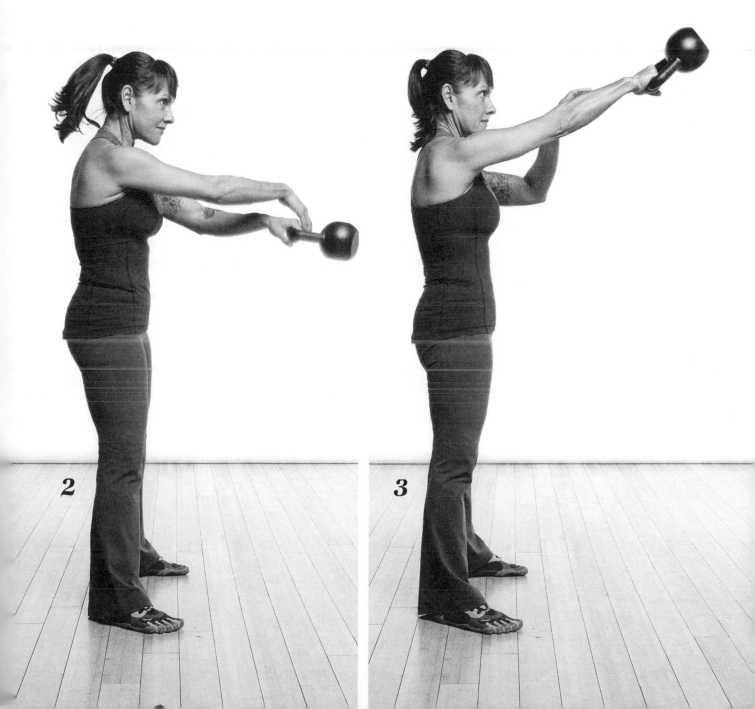

Coach Yourself: Say it out loud as you train: "Swing touch one, swing touch two, swing touch three, swing touch four, switch hands on five, swing touch one, swing touch two, swing touch three, swing touch four, switch back on five."

Since you'll be completing 5 reps on each side, this is how these one-arm swings will appear in the workouts:

5 R/5 L = 5 One-Hand Swings/Touches right (weight in right hand, touching with left hand), switch on five, plus 5 One-Hand Swings/ Touches left, switch back on five, which equals 10 reps.

5 R/5 L × 2 = 5 One-Hand Swings/Touches right, switch on five, plus 5 One-Hand Swings/touches left, switch back on five, repeated twice without rest, which equals 20 reps.

You'll notice that this next batch of workouts is written out a bit differently than the previous workouts. That's because it's time to put all the skills you've learned to work—now you're going to train the kettlebell swing. I write my personal workouts this way because it allows me to see the combinations better and helps me see what comes next with just a quick glance.

The time shown in parentheses after each exercise and number of sets is the total time, meaning it includes both work and rest (see page 131 for more details). These workouts will incorporate the other shorthand terms you've seen, plus another one that indicates a combination of two moves:

+ = the plus sign means you've reached a combination and you should continue right into the next exercise without any rest.

For example, **10 2-hd sw + 5 R/5 L** means you should perform 10 Two-Hand Swings and then go right into 5 One-Hand Swings/Touches right, switch on five, plus 5 One-Hand Swings/Touches left.

The Swing Workouts #1–15: Shorthand Key

Refer back to this key for my shorthand version of all the exercises we'll be using in your workouts.

2-hd sw = Two-Hand swings

5R/5L = 5 One-Hand Swings/Touches right, switch on five, plus 5 One-Hand Swings/Touches left, switch back on five, which equals 10 reps.

5R/5L × 2 = 5 One-Hand Swings, Touches right, switch on five, plus 5 One-Hand Swings, Touches left, switch back on five, repeated twice without rest, which equals 20 reps.

+ = the plus sign means you've reached a combination and you should continue right into the next exercise without any rest.

SW/TR = 1 swing/1 transfer, which equals 2 reps; 10 Swing Transfers equals 20 reps.

TR = transfer

WORKOUT #6

10 2-hd sw × 5 sets (2.5 minutes)

20 2-hd sw × 5 sets (5 minutes)

5 R/5 L × 5 sets (2.5 minutes)

10 2-hd sw × 5 sets (2.5 minutes)

20 2-hd sw × 5 sets (5 minutes)

5 R/5 L × 2 × 5 sets (5 minutes)

10 2-hd sw × 5 sets (2.5 minutes)

Total Workout Time = 25 minutes

WORKOUT #7

10 2-hd sw × 5 sets (2.5 minutes)

5 R/5 L × 5 sets (2.5 minutes)

20 2-hd sw × 5 sets (5 minutes)

5 R/5 L × 2 × 5 sets (5 minutes)

10 2-hd sw + 5 R/5 L × 5 sets (5 minutes)

5 R/5 L + 10 2-hd sw × 5 sets (5 minutes)

Total Workout Time = 25 minutes

Swing Transfers (SW/TR)

Now that you are comfortable switching every 5 reps, you are ready to make the transfers, or switches, happen more frequently. Practice by completing one swing/touch right, and then transferring the bell to your left hand on the next upswing. Repeat on the other side. Now put them together: one swing/touch, one transfer; one swing/touch, one transfer; one swing/touch, one transfer . . . and just keep going! Rest after you get the hang of it. Right now, your rep count doesn't matter; getting the pattern down is what's most important.

Coach Yourself: Say it out loud as you train: "One touch, one transfer, one touch, one transfer."

It's important to point out that for every Swing Transfer, you are completing 2 reps. To make sure you train right and left evenly, all Swing Transfer sets will be at least 20 reps (10 Swing Transfers = 20 reps). Swing Transfers will be indicated as follows in the workouts:

SW/TR = one swing/one transfer, which equals 2 reps;
   10 Swing Transfers equals 20 reps

WORKOUT #8

    10 2-hd sw × 5 sets (2.5 minutes)

    5 R/5 L × 5 sets (2.5 minutes)

    10 SW/TR × 5 sets (5 minutes)

    20 2-hd sw × 5 sets (5 minutes)

    5 R/5 L × 2 × 5 sets (5 minutes)

    10 SW/TR × 5 sets (5 minutes)

    Total Workout Time = 25 minutes

WORKOUT #9

10 2-hd sw × 5 sets (2.5 minutes)

5 R/5 L × 5 sets (2.5 minutes)

10 SW/TR × 5 sets (5 minutes)

10 2-hd sw + 5 R/5 L × 5 sets (5 minutes)

10 2-hd sw + 5 R/5 L + 10 SW/TR × 5 sets (10 minutes)

Total Workout Time = 25 minutes

Transfers (TR)

You are a pro now! Next it's time to practice transferring the bell every rep, but I want you to practice a few sets with one touch first, like you did for the Swing Transfers.

Coach Yourself: Say it out loud as you train: "One swing/touch, swing, transfer at the top, swing, transfer at the top, swing, transfer" . . . and keep going just like that.

Transfers will be indicated as follows in the workouts:

TR = transfer

WORKOUT #10

10 2-hd sw × 5 sets (2.5 minutes)

5 R/5 L × 5 sets (2.5 minutes)

10 2-hd sw + 5 R/5 L × 5 sets (5 minutes)

10 SW/TR × 5 sets (5 minutes)

10 TR × 5 sets (2.5 minutes)

10 2-hd sw + 10 SW/TR + 10 TR × 5 sets (10 minutes)

5 R/5 L × 5 sets (2.5 minutes)

Total Workout = 30 minutes

WORKOUT #11

10 2-hd sw × 2 sets (1 minute)

5 R/5 L × 4 sets (2 minutes)

10 TR × 6 sets (3 minutes)

20 2-hd sw × 2 sets (2 minutes)

5 R/5 L × 2 × 4 sets (8 minutes)

40 TR × 6 sets (12 minutes)

10 2-hd sw × 2 sets (2 minutes)

Total Workout = 30 minutes

WORKOUT #12

10 2-hd sw × 2 sets (1 minute)

5 R/5 L × 2 sets (1 minute)

10 2-hd sw + 5 R/5 L × 2 sets (2 minutes)

10 2-hd sw + 5 R/5 L + 10 2-hd sw + 5 R/5 L × 2 sets (4 minutes)

20 2-hd sw × 2 sets (2 minutes)

5 R/5 L × 2 × 2 sets (2 minutes)

20 TR × 2 sets (2 minutes)

20 2-hd sw + 5 R/5 L × 2 × 2 sets (4 minutes)

20 2-hd sw + 5 R/5 L × 2 + 20 TR × 2 sets (6 minutes)

10 2-hd sw + 5 R/5 L + 10 TR × 2 sets (3 minutes)

10 2-hd sw + 5 R/5 L × 2 sets (2 minutes)

10 2-hd sw × 2 sets (1 minute)

Total Workout = 30 minutes

WORKOUT #13

10 2-hd sw × 2 sets (1 minute)

5 R/5 L × 2 × 2 sets (2 minutes)

10 2-hd sw × 2 sets (1 minute)

20 TR × 2 sets (2 minutes)

10 2-hd sw + 5 R/5 L × 2 sets (2 minutes)

10 2-hd sw + 10 TR × 2 sets (2 minutes)

10 2-hd sw + 5 R/5 L + 10 2-hd sw + 5 R/5 L × 2 sets (4 minutes)

10 2-hd sw + 10 TR + 10 2-hd sw + 10 TR × 2 sets (4 minutes)

10 2-hd sw + 5 R/5 L × 3 sets (1.5 minutes)

10 2-hd sw + 10 TR × 3 sets (1.5 minutes)

10 2-hd sw + 5 R/5 L + 10 TR × 2 sets (3 minutes)

10 2-hd sw + 5 R/5 L + 10 2-hd sw + 10 TR × 2 sets (4 minutes)

10 2-hd sw + 5 R/5 L + 10 2-hd sw + 10 TR × 2 sets (2 minutes)

Total Workout = 30 minutes

Congratulations! You have reached the magic of the two-minute set!

The Magical Two-Minute Set

You have made such a significant accomplishment in getting to this point! You've already arrived at extraordinary; now it's just a matter of pushing yourself to stay on top. I'm sure you have seen an incredible body transformation already, but this final workout will challenge you yet again.

When I first started doing these extended sets, Mark noticed the amazing workout I was getting and named them aerobic threshold sets. He noted that in just two minutes of work, I was experiencing the anaerobic and aerobic benefits of both sprinting and running a marathon.

Both of these final workouts are designed to get you progressively to the two-minute set. At this point, taking equal rest is not important since your cardio endurance has increased and you need less rest. Once you reach 40 reps with a one-minute rest period and you don't need more than a full minute to recover, move on to the next set. Since your rest time could vary, I'm including these last two workouts in a journal format—use them to record rest period changes, as even these will start to shorten. By the time you get to the two-minute set, you will be working a 2:1 work-to-rest ratio.

The Unbeatable Weight-Loss Combo— Anaerobic and Aerobic

By Mark Reifkind

What exactly happens in your body when you perform multiple two-minute sets with the kettlebell? You are working at the crossroads of both the anaerobic (oxygen independent) and the aerobic (oxygen dependent) systems, and getting the best of both. Training with this combination of energy systems is why high intensity kettlebell training was proven to be able to burn 1,200 calories per hour.

When you complete sets that range from fifteen seconds to two minutes, you are doing anaerobic exercise, and the primary source of energy is sugars, which are drawn from both the muscles and the blood. When you complete sets, or perform any intense activity, from two minutes up to twenty minutes, your body pulls more and more energy from fat. Although it might seem better to go longer to draw more energy from fat, training the body to burn sugar for fuel has many advantages. For one, training off of stored muscle sugars (also known as glycogen) creates a demand for the body to store future intake of carbohydrates in the muscles as fuel instead of in the fat.

The relatively short sets (I know—they don't feel short) you're completing also allow for higher training loads and intensities, which work much harder to activate fast-twitch fibers. These are the sprint and strength fibers of the body, and they respond well to harder work and are the ones responsible for increased muscle tone. You train these with anaerobic exercise.

When you perform slow-training, or aerobic, activities like long-distance running, your body uses the slow-twitch or endurance fibers to keep going. While these muscles can perform for a long time, they're stubborn when it comes to increasing in tone or size.

When your kettlebell training reaches the level of two-minute sets, you will be working just short enough to keep a high degree of fast-twitch fibers involved and just long enough to start tapping in to the aerobic system, or slow-twitch fibers. This means you get the best of both worlds: just enough intensity to really develop the muscles and just enough time to really tap in to fat stores as well. You won't find this powerful combination in any other single exercise.

The Swing! WORKOUT #14

Swings	Sets	Rest	Actual Rest
10 2-hd sw	1	15 seconds	
10 R/10 L	1	30 seconds	
5 R/5 L	3	45 seconds	
40 2-hd sw	1	1 minute	
50 TR	1	1.25 minutes	
60 SW/TR	1	1.5 minutes	
5 R/5 L	7	1.75 minutes	
10 R/10 L	4	2 minutes	
5 R/5 L	6	1.5 minutes	
40 SW/TR	1	1 minute	
20 TR	1	30 seconds	
10 2-hd sw	1	DONE!	

Total Workout Time: 18–24 minutes

Notes:

The Swing! WORKOUT #15

Swings	Sets	Rest	Actual Rest
10 2-hd sw	1	15 seconds	
20 2-hd sw	1	30 seconds	
30 2-hd sw	1	45 seconds	
40 2-hd sw	1	1 minute	
50 TR	1	1.25 minutes	
60 SW/TR	1	1.5 minutes	
5 R/5 L × 2	7	1.75 minutes	
10 R/10 L	8	2 minutes	
5 R/5 L	8	2 minutes	
80 SW/TR	1	2 minutes	
80 TR	1	2 minutes	
40 2-hd sw	1	DONE!	

Total Workout Time: 21–28 minutes

Notes:

Continuing Your Progress

Congratulations on all you've accomplished to this point. If you want to continue to strengthen your body and push your results, I invite you to visit my website at giryastrength.com for access to additional kettlebell swing workouts. It's part of who you are now—keep up the amazing work, and know that every day you're swinging, I'm right there with you.

PART THREE

Food

Learning How to Feed You

If your goal is to change your body, then you have to change your eating habits. It sounds obvious, but unless you really take ownership of that change, the transformation won't last. The best way to do this is to connect with the foods you put into your body by learning how to feed yourself.

I'm not referring to just the act of putting food in your mouth—I'm talking about feeding and nourishing your body in a way that makes it flourish and function at its best. If someone else makes and/or prepares your food, then you are not feeding yourself; you are relying on others and blindly trusting them with your most precious possession—your body.

When I first approached creating dietary guidelines for myself, I focused on the goal of creating momentum. Because I was trying to win a bet, I didn't have time to wait around for results—I wanted to jump on the fast track to weight loss. At the same time, I still had the mind of an overeater, and I was not about to starve myself to lose weight. So I came up with two core principles around which I would craft my new way of eating: 1) I had to become intimate with real foods—this meant learning how to cook and connecting to the process of making food for myself (by extension, this also meant no more eating out and ignoring or guessing what ingredients or calories were in my meals), and 2) I had to eat more vegetables than anything else—this would allow me to eat a lot of food while still drastically cutting my calorie consumption.

I'm going to share with you how I took these two principles and turned them into a way to eat for weight loss. Like with your swing workouts, my goal is to inspire you to create a skill and to take responsibility for creating your beautiful, strong, and fit body from the inside out.

Hello, My Name Is Real Food

I changed by body by getting reacquainted with real foods: vegetables, fruits, meats, beans, and grains, you know, those little things called ingredients that you make into meals. If you're living off of packaged meals or fast foods, you're not being fueled by real, live nutrients. When you eat foods that are designed to be preserved, your body has to work really hard to break down all the chemicals just to get to the itty bitty nutritional elements that may be hidden in there, if any exist at all. It's kind of like dumping the contents of a landfill into your body and hoping it finds a few leaves of lettuce in there somewhere. We were not meant to exist on things that only *resemble* real food.

Real food is amazing because it's not calorie dense; it's incredibly, wildly delicious; and there are endless ways to eat it. I didn't start out thinking that way, though. I was a non-cook, but I knew somewhere deep inside that it was important to know how to make foods for myself and for my family. I figured since I loved food so much, I could find a way to love cooking it. I did find a way, and it has honestly turned out to be one of the greatest and most rewarding discoveries of my life.

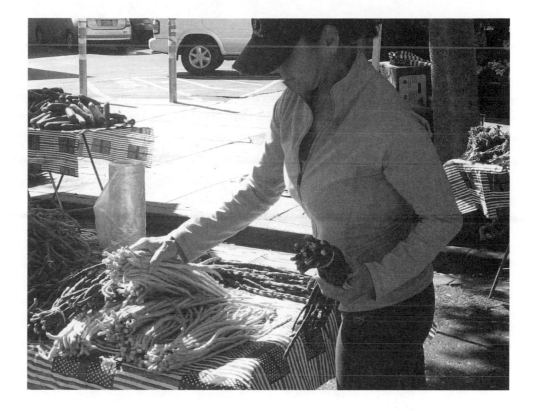

Tracy's Food Rule #1: Diets Work

Why is it said that diets don't work? Seventy percent of the adult female population and 30 percent of all adult males have been on one, but it doesn't seem to matter whether it's the Atkins diet, a low-fat diet, or even a Master Cleanse of only lemon, water, cayenne pepper, and maple syrup; people will try almost anything in a desperate attempt to shed a few pounds—everything except eating right.

A diet stops working when the diet stops, and most dieters choose the wrong diet, and therefore stop dieting. Few dieters maintain their weight loss, and they often end up heavier than they were before they started dieting. So how do you avoid that fate? Don't look at dieting as a vacation from overeating, look at overeating as a vacation from dieting. Learn how to feed yourself, and follow the simple rule of V-First (see page 158).

Understanding Calories

Calories are units of energy, or fuel, that your body uses to function. You burn calories all day long, even when you're just sitting on the couch or brushing your teeth—keeping your bodily systems running burns calories. If you eat more calories than your body naturally burns (your basal metabolic rate), then you gain weight; if you eat less, you lose weight. If you add in exercise, you increase the number of calories burned. And—here's where your body really starts to change—if you burn more calories *and* eat less, well then, your weight loss increases. It is a simple rule; one that's based on pure science. The good news is, science is on your side—it's up to you to start using it to your advantage.

Tracy's Food Rule #2: You Can't Out-Train What You Eat

There is no true equal exchange when it comes to diet and exercise. If you eat a doughnut and then work out an hour later, your body doesn't go straight for those calories like a laser and burn them off. Too often people exercise to make up for what they've eaten, or they eat something and think, "Oh, I'll just burn those calories off!" This is not just a slippery slope; it's the first sign of an avalanche. If you ask people who have successfully maintained their weight loss if they exercise just to burn calories, they will tell you no. When you start swinging a kettlebell, I want you to think about it as creating and improving a skill, and you should look at making your own meals in the same way. When you begin to make your own meals, you aren't just developing the skill of feeding yourself, but you are also establishing a skill to create and re-create, and to consciously choose and bring to life the body you want. I want you to think about feeding your body and not just your mouth (this doesn't mean the foods you'll be eating aren't going to taste great—it's just a thought adjustment that will help you create a more positive and productive relationship with food).

If you're ready to lose weight, it's time to admit that you're eating too much, or in other words, consuming too many calories. Whether it's coming from healthful foods or junk foods is irrelevant at this point. So let's get to work on identifying the number of calories you need to eat to end up at the body weight you were meant to live at; how fast you get there is up to you.

. . . .

Weight Loss vs. Fat Loss

A weight-loss diet is a food-and-eating plan that involves eating fewer calories than you need to maintain your current body weight. If you weigh more than you want to weigh, then you must eat fewer calories than you take in to change this result.

Typically when we lose weight, the loss comes from water, fat, and muscle. There is a popular belief out there that we should want to try and keep all of the muscle and lose only fat. I have news for you: when you are at an unhealthy body weight, you can afford to lose a little bit of all of these components. Worrying about only losing one type of weight is, well, ridiculous at this point. Can you afford to be picky? First things first—get the weight off. All of it. Once you start to lose weight, the majority of the weight you are losing is in fact body fat.

A fat-loss diet, on the other hand, is a diet that focuses specifically on only losing body fat. Talk about scientific. It's usually a high-protein diet that focuses on creating the smallest amount of regular weight loss in the hope of conserving muscle mass. The end goal is to strip the fat to reveal lean muscle. While this may sound like a great goal, it's simply too specific for someone who wants to lose 20 pounds or more. It's even more of a senseless strategy if you're not doing anything to build or keep muscle. So if you're goal is to lose weight, follow the weight-loss principles featured on these pages—they won't fail you (unless you fail them).

. . . .

I'm going to give you a calculation that will provide an approximate number of calories to eat each day based on your goal (assuming your goal is weight loss): take your ideal weight and multiply by 12. This is the approximate number of calories you should be eating each day.

Based on this calculation, if you are a woman who wants to weigh 135 pounds, you would aim to consume about 1,600 calories per day to lose weight; a man wanting to weigh 170 pounds would eat about 2,000 calories. I've estimated these calorie counts based on the lower side of the scale, which you should always do to allow for mistakes—this is what I refer to as a little extra mental insurance.

So here's the question—if you eat the number of calories based on this calculation, will you lose weight? Absolutely. Will you lose weight quickly? Not necessarily. I would say those are numbers you can follow if you want to achieve what I will call average weight loss. If what you want to achieve is *amazing* weight loss, I have some other numbers for you to consider.

Here's why I think 1,600–2,000 calories is simply too high of a range for anyone just starting a weight-loss diet—it's all about momentum. To create some serious momentum toward rapid weight loss, women should consume around 1,200 calories, and men should aim for 1,600. If you aim for these numbers, you will realistically end up consuming 200–400 more calories at least half the time. When I lost 120 pounds, my plan was to eat no more than 1,200 calories a day, except for on my high-calorie day (if I had earned it), but I consumed up to 1,600 calories at times. No one had to tell me that the closer I stayed to 1,200 calories, the faster my results would be—but just in case you need someone to tell you: the closer you stick to 1,200 calories for a woman and 1,600 for a man, the more dramatic your results will be. You know what's great about knowing that? You have no excuse for mediocre results—your results are your responsibility and yours alone, but I'm certainly going to give you every tool in my bag to help you on your way.

Even though keeping an eye on calories is important, I don't plan my meals thinking calories first—I start with nutrients, and then I turn to calories to establish serving sizes. I will go into this in greater detail starting on page 158. However, it does help to think about your meals with general calorie goals. Here's an example of how you could break out your calories for a day:

	1,200-Calorie Day (Women)	1,600-Calorie Day (Men)
Meal 1	350	450
Meal 2	350	450
Meal 3	350	450
Snack	150	250
Total	1,200	1,600

This is a very general guideline that you can manipulate to work for you. You can certainly skip the snack and break that number down into your meals or have larger meals at any point in the day; just aim to hit as close to the total number recommended as possible. And remember that it's likely that you will consume 200–400 undocumented calories—even small bites or sneaky handfuls can add up quickly; how much goes undocumented comes down to your level of motivation to create results.

• •

Tracy's Food Rule #3: You Can Take Weight Off Faster Than You Put It On

You are currently eating enough calories to maintain or increase your body weight, whatever it is. Once you start eating fewer calories, your body will reflect that change in its size—it's pure science. But here's the thing about science: it doesn't operate on emotions, and it doesn't understand fairness; it knows only numbers. This means if you make small changes in your calorie consumption, then you will see small changes in your body weight. If instead you make big changes in your daily calorie consumption, you will see big changes. Even better—if you make big changes quickly, this will produce big changes quickly! So what are you waiting for?

• •

Meal Composition 101

Every good-tasting dish starts with ingredients that balance and complement one another; knowing how and what ingredients to combine to achieve this balance is what makes a good, or even great, cook. All professional chefs create dishes and meals with composition in mind, but you don't have to be a professional to put this knowledge to use in your own kitchen.

Learning and focusing on the concept of composing meals is the key to making lasting changes in your diet for weight loss and maintenance. Taking this approach will help you automatically develop the habits of making better nutritional food choices.

When you think about most common dishes, the protein component plays the lead role, and everything else complements or plays off of the flavors of the protein. The carbohydrate often comes next on the list, and many times a dish stops there. Some well-known meals that follow this order are: steak and potatoes, spaghetti and meatballs, pot roast (beef stew) and rice, fried chicken and biscuits, hot dog on a bun—you get the picture . . . it's just a meat with a starchy carbohydrate. The last element to be considered is the lowly vegetable—maybe a small green salad, steamed broccoli and cauliflower, or microwaved frozen green beans and carrots (since this is the standard experience of vegetables, it's no wonder we go out for burritos and buckets of Chinese food). To top it off, we've practically made cheese its own food group by adding extra to just about every meal at breakfast, lunch, or dinner. This is no way to eat if you have any interest in health, let alone if you have the desire to lose weight and develop a strong and toned body.

The mistake we've been making is leading with the calorie-dense ingredients, like carbs, fats, and protein, instead of the lowest calorie, yet nutrient-dense ingredients: vegetables. I'm going to have you approach your meals in an entirely different order using a strategy that allows you to eat a lot of food with few calories. I call it the V-First approach. This means when you think about your meal composition, you always think *vegetables first*. You will create your meals in this order of priority:

- **Vegetables** (non-starchy)

- **Protein**

- **Fats**

- **Simple and Complex Carbs** (including starchy vegetables)

When you take this order into consideration first, and then use calories as a guide for your serving sizes, no foods are off limits.

Vegetables—A Bigger Plate with Fewer Calories

When it came to changing my diet, volume was a top priority, which I discovered came down to a reordering of the standard way of eating. I knew I wanted to continue to eat a lot of food so I wouldn't feel deprived in any way, and the only way I could do that was to not limit vegetables, the lowest calorie-dense food of all. Little did I know that this simple bit of reorganization would give me so much more than weight loss. It turns out vegetables are highly nutritious and have incredibly satisfying flavor potential.

To make sure I wasn't setting myself up for failure, I set some parameters for my unlimited vegetables rule: first, they weren't entirely undocumented—at the end of each day, I would count all consumed nonstarchy vegetables as having a total of 100 calories; and second, I had to count starchy vegetables for their full calorie value (since the starchy vegetables have a higher carbohydrate content, you'll find them listed them under the carb section; see page 171). You can eat as much as you want of the following vegetables each day, but be sure to count them as 100 calories:

Asparagus

Bell peppers (red, yellow, green)

Broccoli

Brussels sprouts

Cabbage, all varieties

Cauliflower

Carrots

Chard

Celery

Chile peppers, all varieties

Cucumber

Eggplant

Fennel

Green beans

Leafy greens, all varieties (kale, collards, mustard, turnip, beet)

Lettuce, all varieties, including radicchio

Mushrooms

Onions, all varieties (leeks, scallions, shallots)

Summer squashes, all varieties (pattypan, crookneck, zucchini)

Tomatoes (actually a fruit, but listed here for simplicity)

· ·

Not Your Mama's Salad

A salad is not iceberg lettuce, a few unripe tomato slices, and a giant glob of blue cheese—at least not the salads you're going to eat. I'm going to teach you a completely new way of creating salads that are bursting with layers of flavor and texture and are topped with satisfying dressings that don't drown out the flavors of your food. You're going to discover vegetables that are peppery, sweet, savory, and fresh—foods that fill up your bowl and your belly (without filling it out). Not to mention, they're certain to please your taste buds. So keep an open mind when you get to my salad recipes on page 209—the salad has officially been reinvented.

· ·

What you'll discover is that these vegetables are filling and satisfying when you prepare and cook them with the right seasoning and flavors— be adventurous and have fun when you start cooking, and don't be afraid to try new food and flavor combinations.

Here's an example of the vegetables I eat daily:

- 2 cups of fresh spinach, blended into a smoothie

- 4 cups of mixed greens, shredded cabbage, carrot, onion, jalapeño, and cilantro

- 2 cups of veggies (excluding potatoes) as the base for a soup or chili, with all veg scraps going into homemade stocks

- At least a handful of celery, carrot, and broccoli stalk sticks

If you can't tell, that's not only a lot of veggies; it's a lot of food! I promise—you are not going to feel hungry when you start eating like this.

Tracy's Food Rule #4: Flavor Saves

If you steam your veggies, especially ones like brussels sprouts and cauliflower that can have a bitter flavor, you are unlikely to enjoy them. Instead, try roasting them—roasted vegetables are great on their own or in a salad. To roast vegetables, preheat your oven to 400°F. Then, prep 1 to 3 cups of your selected vegetable (if you're using a starchy vegetable, like winter squash, be sure to count the calories) and add 1 tablespoon of olive oil to them, tossing to cover the vegetables as best you can. Sprinkle with salt and pepper, and place in the oven for 30–40 minutes, or until desired doneness. You can also add a squeeze of lemon juice once they're done for added flavor. I want you to think of olive oil, lemon, salt, and pepper as your new best friends. Olive oil adds depth and flavor, lemon adds brightness, a little salt will bring the flavor of foods to the forefront, and pepper adds a kick of spice.

I recommend picking up some sea or kosher salt for your cooking—you'll notice a big difference between these and iodized salts. Do a side-by-side taste test and you will understand what I mean. Besides taste, most cooks use kosher salt because the larger flakes stick to foods and you actually use less. You want your foods to be flavorful, not salty. As every good cook knows, salt enhances the flavors of food, but too much of it can be counterproductive to your goal of weight loss since it causes your body to retain water.

Protein

A lot of people have a problem getting enough protein in their daily meals, but they may not realize why. It's not because it's difficult to prepare proteins or to work them into meals—it's because we have been conditioned to grab the carbs first. We eat cereal, bagels, scones, and so on for breakfast. For lunch, it's a cheeseburger and fries; a burrito made with a tortilla, beans, rice, and a little bit of meat, cheese, and sour cream; pizza, which is again bread, cheese, and a salty meat; or a big, fat sandwich that's mostly bread. Dinner is usually the same—a pile of mashed potatoes with a steak, or maybe a giant bowl of pasta with a few pieces of chicken or ground beef.

Of course, if you go out to eat at a restaurant, you will be eating not only the main course meal but also the basket of chips or the half loaf of bread you started off with on the table. It's no surprise then that people aren't hungry for protein—they're stuffed with filling carbs, most of which have little to no nutritional value. This is why it is so important to learn how to feed yourself instead of relying on restaurants or prepackaged meals. It's time to stop trusting someone else with the job of taking care of your body—you can do so much better.

When you get into the practice of feeding yourself, you'll discover the protein element comes easily. Here's what is on your protein list:

Beef

Chicken and turkey

Cottage cheese

Eggs

Lamb

Pork

Seafood

Cottage cheese is the only dairy in the protein category. This is because it's the only form of dairy that has more protein than it does fat or carbs. All types of dairy have protein, carbs, and fats, but the proportions vary, which is why you'll find them in different categories. For example, you'll see cream and whole milk are considered fats, but low-fat and non-fat milks are listed as carbs because they're mostly lactose, or milk sugar. In keeping with my preference for whole foods and my order of nutrient priority, I will always opt to have the protein and/or fat versions (cottage cheese, cream, or whole milk) during a day, rather than the carbohydrate one (low-fat or non-fat milk).

I list seafood as a protein option, but I personally don't eat a lot of it for a couple reasons. The first is that seafood does not fill me up. The second is based on pure convenience. I like to buy seafood fresh and cook it up the same day to eat, but since I do the bulk of my food prep and cooking so early in the morning, that just doesn't work. Plus, seafood only keeps for two days, and I prefer to stock my fridge with meals that last a bit longer. There are exceptions, like frozen shrimp and salmon burgers, which are easier to buy in advance, but it's just too much extra effort for me on a regular basis. However, seafood is one of the fastest foods to cook, and it tastes great with minimal ingredients, so if you can make it work for you at home, it can be an excellent protein option.

Most proteins are easy to prepare, and these days you can even find ready-made options that you can add to meals. Whether you make it yourself or buy it, you can get four to six meals out of a roasted chicken, a pound of ground meat, or a dozen eggs. I recommend buying full-fat (non-lean) cuts of meat for the flavor, but just be sure to count the calories in the portion you've eaten.

Here's an example of what your protein consumption could look like over the course of a day:

- ½ to 1 cup of cottage cheese (100–200 calories)

- 4 ounces chicken or pork tenderloin in a salad (171–185 calories)

- 4 ounces beef, lamb, or pork (185–300 calories), which I would normally add to a soup, stew, or chili

If you are a vegetarian and you are overweight, I want you to apply the same principle to your meals—put veggies first, and your calories will fall into place. Even though I eat meat, I'm certain I eat more vegetables than most vegetarians. A lot of vegetarians are really just non-meat eaters because they often base their meals around carbs and cheese. Meals like bagels with cheese, nachos with cheese, and grilled cheese sandwiches may not have any meat, but they're certainly not healthful. True vegetarians eat vegetables more than anything else, which means it's highly unlikely they are overweight. If you are a vegetarian who doesn't need to lose weight, but you want to know how to change your body, my advice remains the same: vegetables first (and of course, kettlebell workouts).

Fats in Your Food
(How to Make a Little Go a Long Way)

For years after I decided to change my body, I rarely ate cheese, but somehow I didn't even notice it was missing. The reason for this is that when I composed my meals, cheese never made the priority list. This doesn't mean you can't eat cheese—if you want to eat 1,200 calories of cheese and call it a day, go right ahead (though I'm sure it will be a one-time binge considering how you'll feel afterward).

Even if you want to eat just a little cheese, keep in mind that its proportion of fat is higher than its other nutritional qualities, and don't forget the high sodium content. This means it has a high calories-to-volume ratio (fat has more calories per ounce than carbs or proteins). I prefer to use my fats in a way that benefits or dresses up my vegetables. By using olive oil to sauté, roast, or grill veggies, or by adding it to a large salad as part of a dressing, you will satisfy your palate with a bit of fat without overdoing it.

Fat is not the enemy. In fact, it's important to keep fat calories in your diet for several reasons: they provide energy; they add flavor and texture to keep foods from becoming dry and bland; they help absorb the fat-soluble vitamins D, E, and A; and they provide a greater sense of satisfaction, which helps prevent hunger, whereas cutting fats too much can trigger cravings or binge eating.

So how do you keep fats in your diet without consuming all your calories for the day? Well, the good news is that if you pick the right forms of fat, a little can go a long way. I begin every cooked dish with a fat, usually in the form of one tablespoon of olive oil. Salad dressings are a base of fat and acid; the fat is usually in the form of olive oil, to which I add something acidic, such as vinegar or lemon juice.

Let's take a look at some other fats. Dairy fats, besides cheese, are: butter, cream, half-and-half, and whole milk (not low-fat or non-fat). Then there are the nut butters, like peanut butter, almond butter, and so on. And a couple sneaky fats to remember are whole nuts and avocados, which a lot of people label as healthful fats. I'm not going to get into healthful fats because when you are trying to lose weight, you should limit *all* fats to a certain percentage of your daily calories.

Fats are roughly 100–120 calories per tablespoon or serving size, so based on a 1,200–1,600 daily allotment of calories, you should have about 150–300 fat calories per day. Does this seem like a lot or a little to you? If it seems like a lot, then you must have no idea how much fat you are consuming right now, which I'm sure has contributed to any issues you have with weight. You will discover, as I did, that a large part of changing your diet is about plain and simple awareness—especially if you've been relying on others to make meals for you, you have no idea what you've been eating. Here's the breakdown of my daily fat consumption:

- 1 tablespoon of cream (52 calories)

- 1 tablespoon mayonnaise or olive oil in dressing (57–120 calories)

- 1 ounce of nuts or 2 tablespoons of peanut butter (about 185 calories)

When I use oil (up to 2 tablespoons) to start a soup, stew, or chili, I don't count the calories because it gets distributed significantly throughout the whole batch, and each portion has very little oil.

Carbs

When most people think of carbohydrates, they think of potatoes, bread, and chips, but in reality, carbohydrates exist in various forms and amounts in almost every type of food. I think it's easiest to look at carbs in two categories: simple and complex. Sugar, honey, fresh fruit, dried fruit, fruit juice, low-fat milk products (because they're mostly milk sugar), and alcohol fall into the simple carb category. Complex carbs include foods like rice, beans, pasta, oats, grains, flour, and starchy vegetables like peas, potatoes, squash, and corn. I'm going to give you an overview of the different types of carbohydrates and share with you my strategies for being smart about your carb selection.

Simple Carbs

For our purposes, simple carbs will include: sugar (all forms), fresh fruit, dried fruit, fruit juice, low-fat milk products, and alcohol. These carbohydrates are called simple because they have a basic molecular structure, which means they break down into glucose quickly. This allows for them to become usable energy very quickly, which can be good if you need the energy. If you don't need it—and chances are you don't because you probably have enough stored energy (fat)—then it converts to stored energy, or more fat.

I have always had a sweet tooth, so when I first started creating dietary principles for myself, I knew I had to cater to my natural taste cravings in some way. One of the best tricks I discovered is to incorporate sweetness into my meals by adding something like honey or brown sugar to a dressing or marinade. This way you get the flavor satisfaction without all the calories you would consume if you ate, say, six chocolate chip cookies (my favorite former dessert from McDonald's). I make marinades and dressings that are composed of fat (oil), salt (soy sauce), sugar (honey or brown sugar), and some kind of acid (vinegar, or lemon or lime juice), and seasoning like spices and herbs. I've found that giving a grilled or broiled piece of meat or fish a touch of sweet flavor or eating a delicious, dessert-like salad can stave off a future sugar craving.

When it comes to what type of sugar to use, I recommend real ingredients rather than artificial. This means choosing options like brown sugar, white sugar, honey, and molasses. Artificial sweeteners, such as aspartame and sucralose, can be hundreds of times sweeter than real sugars and therefore can distort your palate as you work toward transforming it. Over-flavored and processed foods are not conducive to retraining your taste buds to crave fresher, healthier foods.

For me, having a sweet tooth also means having a fondness for fruit, which can be just as tempting to overdo as candy. The problem with fruit is its high sugar content—it can be a high-calorie trap, so it's important to monitor your serving sizes and make smart selections. For example, I love grapes, so much so that I can still eat a whole pound in one sitting (around 300 calories). Because of this, one of the rules I created for myself is to only buy the amount of grapes that I can eat based on the number of calories I want to consume. That means I'll typically buy ⅓ pound of grapes, which is approximately 100 calories. Another tip is to buy only fruits that have a higher fiber content and are therefore more filling. For example, an apple with the skin on (95 calories for a medium one) is one of my favorite snacks, and I can tell you I've never been tempted to eat two—they are definitely my number-one fruit choice.

Use common sense, though, and know that an extra-large piece of fruit is going to have twice as many calories as a small one. Even when it comes to something you might think of as healthful, don't try to get away with anything—stick to counting the calories in your foods. As for fruit juices, I recommend skipping them; it's better to eat your calories than to drink them. If you have to have some flavorful liquid, like juice or soda, start to

• •

Tracy's Food Rule #5: Healthful Choice? Not So Fast

Some starchy fruits are more calorie dense and will make your total calorie count higher than you think. How can fruit be bad? How can any fresh food be bad? Too much of a good thing is still too much. No matter what the nutritional value, eating too many calories will contribute to weight gain. Some fruits—such as bananas, mangoes, grapes, and cherries—can add up quickly in calories mostly because you are more likely to overeat them. Keep a close eye on your consumption of these fruits!

• •

wean yourself from the full-strength versions by adding water to juice or sparkling water to soda. Continue diluting it until you get to at least a 50:50 ratio. This way, you get the flavor without the excess calories.

Dried fruits are concentrated sugar, and the calories reflect this. Be extra careful of dried fruits with added sugar; a lot of times you will find sugar has been added to dried varieties of cranberries, pineapple, and mango, so just be sure to check the label. You can use dried fruits like raisins in your salads, trail mix, or even soups—I love them in cauliflower soup, with lentils, and as an addition to savory dishes to give it a delicious sweet-and-savory combination. The calories add up quickly, though, so don't go overboard—raisins have around 33 calories per tablespoon.

Non-fat and low-fat milk also fall into the category of simple carbohydrates because they're mostly lactose, or milk sugar. I recommend selecting the forms of dairy that are considered protein or fats (half-and-half, heavy whipping cream) before these options; this way, you get to enjoy the richer, more satisfying flavors.

Wine and other alcoholic drinks are carbs, and if you consume them, you must count the calories just like with everything else. When I first modified my diet, I didn't drink any alcohol, and for over three years it

∙ ∙

Tracy's Food Rule #6: Eat Sweet Without Sabotage

I never cut sugar completely from my diet because I knew it was a restriction that wouldn't work for me, and because I don't view sugar as some sort of enemy. There are creative and smart ways to satisfy your sweet tooth without sabotage. For example, when you use dressings or marinades with a hint of sweetness, you can satisfy a sweet craving—it may take some time to reeducate your palate, but once you do, you'll discover that a little sugar goes a long way. I have sweetness in my smoothies in the form of sugar, honey, or maple syrup. I like sweet, I like sugar, and I'm not going to apologize for it! Enjoy sweetness, but just be smart about it by ensuring you measure your quantities and count your calories.

∙ ∙

never came into play—I just wasn't willing to spend 150–200 calories on a glass of wine, not even on my high-calorie day (see page 172 for more on the high-calorie day). However, I recently started to enjoy a glass or two of red wine almost every night, but I always figure the calories into my daily allotment. If you choose to drink alcohol, just be sure to do the same.

Here's a quick glance at how your daily simple carbohydrate consumption could shape up—you'll notice it's not a lot, but like I mentioned, once you've trained your palate to appreciate fresh, real foods, measured sweetness will be plenty satisfying:

- 1 tablespoon of raisins or 2 prunes (33–40 calories)

- 1 medium apple, or 1 cup of grapes (95–104 calories)

- 1 tablespoon of sugar in a smoothie, oatmeal, or salad dressing (46 calories)

Complex Carbs

The other type of carbohydrate is the complex carb, which includes starchy vegetables, rice, beans, pasta, oats, grains, and flour. These foods can be calorie dense, so be sure to familiarize yourself with the calorie counts of your favorite staples. Complex carbs are calorie dense and tend to make me feel bloated, which is why they're the last category I consider in my meal composition. Most complex carbs will create some type of bloat because they have the potential to hold up to four times their weight in water. Pay attention to how your body feels the day after you eat them so you can make adjustments accordingly (since your goal is to lose weight, feeling bloated is not exactly a welcome experience).

The starch-heavy vegetables you should count as carbs are: beets; peas; winter squashes, such as butternut, acorn, and spaghetti squash; parsnips; all types of potatoes; corn; and plantains.

Here's the breakdown of what your daily complex carbohydrate consumption could look like:

- ½ cup dry oats (150 calories) or ¾ cup cooked spaghetti (132 calories)

- 1 cup butternut squash (82 calories) or ¾ cup cooked split peas, beans, barley, rice, or lentils in a stew or chili (145–175 calories)

And there you have it—you're now armed with a simple strategy with which to approach your meals. Start with vegetables first, then proteins, fats, and finally carbohydrates, and you will make a smart plate that fuels your body without filling it out. Keep in mind that the daily consumption examples I listed within each category are meant to be used as a general guideline—mix and match these items and aim for 1,200 calories if you're a woman, 1,600 calories if you're a man. The closer you stick to these numbers, the faster the weight will fall off.

Your Oats, Not Mine

Oatmeal works for me. I love it and look forward to eating oatmeal, and it's consistently been the one "carb-only" meal I eat. Here's what's great about it: 1) you get a huge serving from just ½ cup of dry oats, 2) you can make it sweet or savory, and 3) it will keep you regular. I often have oatmeal for dinner because it leaves me feeling satisfied and sleepy. Plenty of people out there will tell you that you have to eat steel-cut oats for it to be beneficial, but I don't discriminate between Cream of Wheat, hot multigrain cereals, steel-cut oats, or plain instant oatmeal. While the nutritional content may differ slightly between these various types, what's most important is that it makes you happy and it's something you look forward to. Believe me, it's not your oatmeal selection that will keep you fat or make you gain weight—it's everything else you end up eating when you don't enjoy the foods on your diet. This is your diet and no one else's, so eat the foods you love, but just do it wisely.

The Argument for the High-Calorie Day

You may have heard that your body can adapt to eating fewer calories by slowing its metabolism—it's true, and when that happens, you can hit a plateau or actually gain weight while eating a reduced-calorie diet. Imagine that nightmare. So how do you ensure this doesn't happen? You spike your calories once a week with a lovely concept called the high-calorie day (I don't like to always refer to it as a cheat day because that suggests it's a bad thing). Here's the tricky part—you are only allowed the high-calorie day *if* you first meet your weight-loss goal during the week. How do you ensure you meet your weight-loss goal each week? You stick as close as you can to the calorie range of 1,200 calories a day for women, and 1,600 calories a day for men.

It's important to approach the high-calorie day with a little uncommon common sense. I know how much food people can eat when they're told that they can eat whatever they want, nonstop, from morning to night, pedal to the metal, whole hog literally for one full day—and it's really not necessary to go on a twenty-four-hour binge in order to feel you've had a break from your eating guidelines. Two hours is plenty.

Let's think in terms of one of my other favorite activities: shopping. Have you ever wondered what it would be like to win a shopping spree? You know, the kind where the store gives you a huge shopping basket and let's you run riot for maybe two minutes? Do you think the store would ever let you go crazy for an entire day? You'd absorb all their profits and then some. Just like that store, I know better than to tell an overeater to spend the whole day feeding their face. This is why it's important to approach your high-calorie day with a few parameters.

When I first created principles for how I was going to eat, the rule I set for my cheat day was that I had to earn it by meeting my weekly weight-loss goal. It was pretty simple for me because I was eating foods I loved in order to lose weight; it wasn't hard. Since my husband and I had a weekly date night, I decided to cheat on that night because I wanted it to be free of any restrictions. I ate everything I wanted to—and lots I didn't necessarily want to (like on a shopping spree, you just start grabbing whatever you can get your hands on).

Eventually, I got better at picking and choosing the foods I wanted to treat myself to on that one night. Then, the day after, I would lower my calories to a more precise 1,200, and I was pretty strict on this one day, more so than any other. The result: I always lost whatever weight I might have gained from the high-calorie day. That way I was ready to start the next week energized and motivated all over again. I'm telling you—it's worth it, and it will keep your momentum driving forward at full speed.

This type of calorie cycling isn't just a trick I made up; it's a common practice in the sport of bodybuilding. Bodybuilders figured out very early in the eighties that consistently lowering their caloric intake would stop their fat loss efforts since the body adapts to the lower intake by slowing the metabolism. Spiking their calories served two purposes: the first was to remind the body that it wasn't going to starve, which would keep its metabolism high; the second was for psychological reasons—allowing this day off made it easier to stick to their diet throughout the week. Trust me, you are going to look forward to that free day. Just remember, you have to earn it.

So let's review the rules for the high-calorie day:

- **Weight loss is essential.** If you did not lose weight during week, you do not get a cheat day. Why? Because you've obviously been overeating enough during the week. One of the reasons for a cheat day is to get a break from the mental stress of calorie restriction, but if you haven't truly been eating within your calorie range, then you don't need a mental break. You can either expect results or hope for them—let your actions create your expectations.

- **Choose one mealtime or "two hours to devour."** This time frame should fall on the same day each week (the body craves and responds well to consistency). Yes, it's called a high-calorie day, but you really don't need an entire day to satisfy all your pent-up cravings. Get your fill in a set period of time; then aim to eat normally the rest of the day, whether it's in the morning or evening.

- **Follow up your cheat day with a low-calorie day.** I know that sticking with the low-calorie day after the high-calorie day strategy helped keep me motivated because I never had to see the number on the scale go up, but it's not an essential rule to follow—just do the best you can with it. You've got the rest of the week to catch up, and scientifically you really didn't do much damage, if any at all, to your weight loss; in fact, you are preventing damage by spiking your calories. If you see a weight gain, it's probably just those carbs (we both know you're going to have carbs on your cheat day) holding onto water. If you want to avoid even a temporary weight gain, follow the high-calorie day with a low-calorie day closer to around 1,000 calories (1,250–1,300 calories for men).

Food Journaling

As you get ready to change your daily eating habits, I want to emphasize how important it is to track what you're eating in a food journal. The best way to approach the idea of tracking calories is to simply look at it as data. If you don't want to educate yourself on the facts of your daily calorie consumption, then you already know the problem and are afraid to face it, and you're probably not truly ready for change. Just like stepping on a scale, though, it can be liberating to take responsibility. Looking at the nutritional information on the packages of all the foods you choose will become first nature, and that's not bad. Becoming an expert on food is fun; make a game out of it!

You'll find a blank food journal in the Appendices (see page 239) that you can copy and use each day. I recommend you keep a running total throughout the day, which means carrying a little notebook with you or, if you have a smartphone, downloading one of the many apps now available for tracking foods and calories. A couple of examples of my own food journals are shown on the following pages.

When I first started keeping track of what I was eating, I did it at the end of each day from memory, but I have found it much easier to journal a few times throughout the day, although not necessarily right after you've eaten. The important point is to jot it down soon enough that you don't forget (accidentally or purposefully).

While it's important to track everything, I don't want you to treat food journaling like your taxes or to feel like it's your judge and jury. Think of it more like scientific data you've collected on your body—you'll be able to understand what foods make you feel sluggish, heavy, or bloated, what foods make you feel light and energized, and what flavors really please your palate.

Do you have to be militant with your tracking? No. I believe in order for it to become a consistent activity, it must not feel like homework. I often guess a bit on the high side, and I don't list literally every single calorie that passes my lips. I don't count single bites of stuff (unless it's followed by another), nor do I count small portions like two almonds. I have a Misc. category where I list a guess between 50 and 100 calories based on that particular day. Instead of writing something precise like "10 carrot sticks = 8 calories," I'll just list "handful of carrot sticks" at the end of the day along with all other "unlimited" veggie calories and count them as 100. Be honest with yourself and allow your food journal to become as close to an accurate record of your calorie consumption as possible, but don't let it take the fun out of eating.

The Swing! **DAILY EATING JOURNAL**		
DATE: 3/26		
Meal 1:	Veggies: n/a	Time: 11:30 A.M.
	Protein: ½ cup, whole milk (73 calories)	
	Fat: n/a	
	Carbs: ½ cup, old-fashioned oats (150 calories) 1 tablespoon, sugar (45 calories)	
Meal 2:	Veggies: 4 cups, cabbage salad mix	Time: 3:30 P.M.
	Protein: 4 ounces, chicken thigh meat (200 calories)	
	Fat: dressing (150 calories)	
	Carbs: 1 cup, grapes (62 calories)	
Meal 3:	Veggies: onion, carrot, celery, tomato, chard (in chili)	Time: 5:30 P.M.
	Protein: 3 ounces, ground lamb (150 calories)	
	Fat: n/a	
	Carbs: 1 cup, black beans (225 calories)	
Snacks:	1 chocolate sucker (80 calories)	
	Unlimited veggies (100 calories)	
WORKOUT: Activity: 6:00 A.M.: 2-mile walk; 7:15 A.M.: Bikram yoga		
NOTES: Total calories: 1,235		

The Swing!	**DAILY EATING JOURNAL**	
DATE: 3/27		

	Veggies: 4 cups, cabbage salad mix	Time: 11:30 A.M.
Meal 1:	Protein: 4 ounces, chicken thigh meat (200 calories)	
	Fat: dressing (150 calories)	
	Carbs: 1 ounce, raisins (90 calories)	
Meal 2:	Veggies: spinach, tomato, cucumber (smoothie)	Time: 3:30 P.M.
	Protein: 1 cup, cottage cheese (200 calories)	
	Fat: ½ avocado (135 calories)	
	Carbs: n/a	
Meal 3:	Veggies: onion, carrot, celery, chard	Time: 6:30 P.M.
	Protein: 3 ounces, ground lamb (150 calories)	
	Fat: n/a	
	Carbs: 1 cup, black beans (225 calories)	
Snacks:	carrot, celery, and broccoli	Time: 1:00 P.M.
	2 tablespoons, peanut butter (200 calories)	
	Unlimited veggies (100 calories)	

WORKOUT:
Activity: 6:00-6:45 A.M.: kettlebell training; 7:00 A.M.: 2-mile walk

NOTES:
Total calories: 1,450

11

Putting It All into Practice

When I changed my diet and starting cooking for myself, I had just recently learned how to cook by taking some classes at a local gourmet kitchen store. I had never roasted a chicken, grilled a steak, or made a pot of soup. My entire life I had wanted to have this skill, but I didn't grow up in a family where cooking was a priority, let alone something that was taught and passed on. What was the most embarrassing, now that I look back, was that I was trying to raise a family with no experience or knowledge of how to feed them. Now I have the skill to feed them—and myself—well.

You might think you're too busy to cook, but you're not. In this chapter, I'm going to give you some invaluable tips for how to make meal preparation fast and easy. When you apply the simple strategies I've suggested for you here, you'll discover that food preparation happens at a much quicker pace than you're used to. You might even be surprised to discover that cooking, even just cutting vegetables, is a calming and meditative process. I dare you to enjoy it.

Getting into the Rhythm of Cooking

There's no better investment than learning how to cook. I'm not talking about complex recipes or techniques, but everyday skills and methods that anyone can learn quickly and then apply in the kitchen to make cooking simple and fun. It's not complicated, but a little bit of knowledge can go a long way. The more you cook, the easier and more enjoyable it becomes, and just as with any skill, it takes time to develop.

The most valuable foundational lessons I learned when I first started cooking were how to prep foods with a knife and how to set up my kitchen before cooking a meal; knowing these simple strategies helped me transition smoothly into cooking my own meals. Read on to learn how you can integrate these two lessons into your own cooking habits.

Knife Skills

One of the most important foundations of becoming a good cook is learning how to use a knife. You may know how to cut foods, but chances are, unless you prep foods regularly, you're not very fast at it. Practice—that is, just doing it a lot—is the only way that will make it easier and faster to cook your own meals. How do you think Rachael Ray can have so many meals in her 30-Minute Meals repertoire? Because she has the knife skills to get the work done quickly. Prepping correctly will also improve the quality and taste of your foods.

The most important detail to strive for when it comes to cutting and chopping foods is consistency in size. Don't worry if it's not perfect—you'll become more comfortable and proficient in your skills with practice. One simple way to make prepping foods easier is to make sure you are using the right type of knife—I recommend an 8- or 10-inch chef's knife.

Creating confidence in your knife skills takes practice, but the more you cook, the better you'll get. One of my favorite ways to practice and improve my knife skills is to make something known as a mirepoix (mir-pwah), which is a French term used to describe a basic mixture of carrots, onions, celery, and herbs that is sautéed in oil or butter. Virtually every soup and stew recipe starts with mirepoix. There is no better way to hone your knife skills than practicing with this mix. To try it, simply get one small onion, two carrots, and two to three celery stalks. Chop each ingredient into a fine to medium dice, aiming to create uniformity in size and shape. Pick a day to pre-chop mirepoix for a number of dishes that you want to have during the week, and store it in an airtight container in the fridge until you are ready to use it. Once you get in the habit of all the chopping, it doesn't take long, but getting it done ahead of time will make cooking that much faster and easier.

• •

Tracy's Food Rule #7: Chop an Onion a Day

When someone tells me that they don't like onions, I suspect what they really mean is they don't like raw onions, because practically every savory dish you make requires an onion. Cutting an onion correctly is a skill that only develops with practice. First, you cut the onion in half from root to stem. Place the flat side of the cut onion on the cutting board and slice off the stem end (the non hairy side). Here's the trickiest part: make some horizontal cuts toward the root end, but not through the root because the root is what holds the onion together while you cut it. Push the knife forward, away, and then pull toward you as this will make horizontal cutting easier. Now make your vertical cuts, and you've chopped an onion. If you chop an onion each day, you are likely to use it somewhere—in a soup, in a stew, in a pasta sauce. Just an act of making your own meal, even if it is only once a day, will go a long way to cutting your intake of calories. The act of chopping an onion is a first step you can take toward eating right—just like walking, it's an entry point into healthier living because it represents connecting with real foods and flavors. While mastering the skill of chopping an onion (and using it), you will come to appreciate how easy other foods are to chop and prepare.

• •

Everything in Place

There's another phrase in French that I love: *mise en place*. It's a basic concept of cooking that means "everything in place." When you cook, everything goes much smoother if you have all the foods and tools you'll need at the ready. Especially when you're making a recipe for the first time, it is highly recommended that you have all the ingredients you need together, *in one place*, before you start cooking. The most obvious place is your kitchen counter, but if you don't have a lot of space, a side

· ·

The Gateway to Cooking: Ready-Made Foods

I hope I've convinced you and inspired you to make and prepare all of your own foods—I can't emphasize enough how important this step was to making my diet become a lifestyle. If you need a transitional method because you've convinced yourself you have *to purchase ready-made foods, then purchase only foods, not ready-made meals, and put them together—this can be part of your progression toward making your own meals entirely. Even if you opt for ready-made foods, establish the minimum commitment of making and preparing at least one of your three meals.*

The difference between buying ready-made meals and ready-made foods is that the foods require you to be more hands-on, which will move you closer toward cooking for yourself. If you pick up a roasted chicken at the grocery store and add this to a home-prepared salad, you have evolved beyond just picking up an entirely pre-made Chinese chicken salad. Buying the whole salad prepped will not teach you about food preparation, but buying shredded cabbage and adding it to other seasonal veggies will be an entry-level lesson. The more hands on you are, the more satisfied and confident you will become in feeding yourself, and the faster your evolution toward cooking entirely for yourself will take place.

· ·

or kitchen table will do. Once you're ready to start actually making the meal, everything is right in front of you. This will also help you avoid forgetting any ingredients or steps. If you are missing one or two ingredients, don't worry. Just keep on cooking because no matter how it turns out, you'll have practiced, and there's always a way to make something edible. When I have flops in the kitchen, good taste comes second to hot and edible. If you start with fresh ingredients, how bad could it be?

Once you have everything set up, it's time to start chopping, slicing, and dicing. Do this before you even think about turning on the stovetop—unless of course the recipe requires preheating the oven. Since you'll be making a lot of delicious, hearty salads on this plan, you can actually prep a lot of your foods up to a week in advance (see page 209).

Planning Your Meals

Do you know what you're going to eat today? If the answer is no, then you need to get into the practice of planning for your meals and preparing them ahead of time. This is quite possibly *the* most important part of establishing who or what dictates your future health and body weight—is it going to be chance or you? Chance hasn't worked so far, so it's time to try preparation instead. I can tell you what I'm going to eat today, because there isn't a week that goes by when I don't know what my main meals are going to be or that I don't have them already prepared in advance. I wouldn't want it any other way.

The simplest and most efficient way to approach eating each week is to choose the same meals to have for at least four days out of seven. (If you look at what you're eating now, you're probably eating the same half a dozen meals or so on a rotation; you're just eating the wrong meals.) Prepping the same meals alleviates the need to make decisions and choices, and it frees you up to focus on other important tasks during your day. This habit is crucial to establishing long-term weight-loss success. Ask most people who have never had extra body weight what they eat every day, and more times than not, they will tell you they eat basically the same foods. During these past six years of maintaining my weight loss, I'm convinced the one time I gained back 20 pounds was because I broke this habit. Looking back over food journals, I identified what had changed, and as soon as I went back to a routine menu, the weight practically fell off. Our bodies like consistency; in fact, they thrive off it.

There's a world of choices out there, and you can't possibly eat everything, although you've probably spent plenty of time trying—I know I did. It's not about focusing on what you can't have, or what you think you're missing out on, because the truth is that nothing is off limits. When you focus on learning how to compose your meals in order of nutritional priority, you will feel more satisfied than ever. You'll be eating plenty of food throughout the week, and remember you always have your high-calorie day not too far off in the distance. Don't worry that you are missing out; all you will truly be missing out on is getting, or staying, fat!

. . . .

Tracy's Food Rule #8: You Can Eat Well on Any Budget

You don't have to buy expensive organic fruits and vegetables to lose weight or to get healthy. At one time, I tried to buy everything organic and found that it made food prep stressful, not only because I had to schedule extra time for tracking down what I needed from different farmers' markets and grocery stores, but also because it added too many more questions than I could handle when it came to selecting foods: Is this local enough? Does this one have more chemicals than that one? Eventually, I just had to relax because I was overcomplicating something I loved. If you have the time and money to visit your local farmers' markets, I highly encourage you to do it, but don't create more rules for your eating habits than you have to for success.

. . . .

I love to use Sunday as my prep day. Sunday is a great day to go to the farmers' markets or the grocery store, and it's a great day to dedicate to your personal well-being. A word of caution: *never, ever try to do food prep when you are hungry*. I recommend doing it at a time of day when food is least tempting, or even about twenty minutes after you've eaten a meal. I do almost all of my food prep before seven in the morning, or even first thing when I wake up at four. I never want to eat anything that early, and I'm barely able to bring myself to taste for seasoning adjustments. This has proven to be a brilliant strategy for me because I also have the most energy right away in the morning and I'm not tempted to snack or munch on anything I'm preparing. There are no rules that say you have to do your food prepping or cooking in the evenings.

Shopping List Regulars

There are a number of items that you should have in your refrigerator or pantry at all times. When you're ready to head for the grocery store, refer to this list of must-haves:

- Salad vegetables: cabbage, lettuce, spinach, or any of your favorite greens

- Fats: olive oil, mayo

- Pick your protein: chicken, beef, pork, lamb, eggs

- Base and broth vegetables: onions, celery, and carrots (mirepoix)

- Acidic ingredients: lemons, limes for juice

- Dairy: yogurt, cottage cheese

- Fruit: apples or dried fruit

- Sweeteners: sugar or honey

- Grains/legumes: beans, rice, oats

- Spices: salt and pepper

On your prep day, you should shred, chop, and dice your salad vegetables and make any dressings you plan to use. You can also cook proteins separately or in big batches of soup and stews. Pre-portioning your meals is just as important as pre-cooking them. Be sure to stock up on containers to portion out servings as you make them—this is a huge time-saver later in the week! It's especially important to pre-portion snacks. One unmeasured handful of something inevitably leads to another, which leads to another. By pre-portioning snacks into serving sizes, this gives you a cutoff reminder and you are more likely to stop after one . . . or maybe two.

You'll discover that some foods might get a big soggy or change consistency if you prepare them too far in advance, such as certain salad greens, breads (which you should limit anyway), and some grains, as well as dried fruits, which can swell up like balloons. Keep in mind that this is a learning process, and make notes about what components to keep separate for the first couple of days.

When you eat at a restaurant, especially a fast-food restaurant, how do you think they make the food so fast? They're certainly not chopping your ingredients when you order your meal. The kitchen staff gets there hours in advance to start cleaning, chopping, dicing, measuring, pre-roasting, grating, prepping, and anything else they can do in advance to make their job easier when it comes to serving your meal. Sure, they might have a few more people in their kitchen than you do, but that doesn't mean you can't borrow the strategy. Like a restaurant, you want to be ready to create great meals in just a short amount of time. You can also create your own soup and salad bars by taking out a bunch of your prepped foods to make a meal—it's just as fun and simple at home as it is at a restaurant or grocery store (plus, it's better tasting).

If you haven't established a close relationship with your freezer, get ready to do so now. So many foods freeze beautifully, such as soups, stews, and chilis, and there are several other types of food that freeze and thaw out perfectly well. You can freeze individual portions of proteins, like diced chicken breast for salads, or portions of cooked grains, beans, and rice, which can be added to salads or soups.

It's important to start seeing just about everything as reheatable and re-eatable. If you think you don't like leftovers, it's time to change the way you think. Otherwise you are going to spend a lot more time in the kitchen or at the bank depositing your paycheck to pay for "freshly" made foods each day.

If you are already fast and efficient at some of your favorite recipes, then by all means, make it as easy as possible on yourself by continuing to make these meals. Just be sure to go to a website like www.calorieking.com to calculate the total number of calories in the dish, and then divide by number of servings. To be absolutely on target with your calories, you could also invest in a small nutritional scale. If a dish is high calorie, between 350–450 per single serving, you can always use my technique for expanding foods by adding a small portion to a salad or soup (see page 196). This way you'll eat a filling meal and still be able to stick to your calorie goal for the day.

When to Eat

My eating schedule has been highly successful for me, and it's based on a proven timing method that's been around for decades. While it may seem a bit unconventional at first, I encourage you try it—remember, what you've been doing hasn't worked, so anything is worth a shot.

I define breakfast as the first meal of the day, and I usually eat my first meal around eleven A.M. It may not sound that late, but I wake up at four A.M., which means I don't eat until seven hours after I've gotten up. Everyone from expert to ordinary person has heard an opinion or has an opinion about when and if to eat breakfast. What I'm going to tell you is what works for me now and what worked for me when I lost 120 pounds.

First thing in the morning, I have coffee with full-fat cream, which keeps my blood sugar levels from dropping. The fat in the cream helps prevent hunger from brewing by only minimally stimulating insulin levels. Insulin is a transport hormone that is generated when you eat to help move the energy from the food into your cells for use. It's produced whenever you eat anything, but your pancreas secretes it like crazy when you eat carbs. Carbs drive up your blood sugar faster, which results in you feeling hungry. Here's a quick scenario of how this works: if you eat a bunch of simple carbs or sugar, your blood sugar rapidly goes up and your body secretes insulin to move that blood sugar into your muscle cells or fat cells, which leaves your blood sugar low. When your blood sugar drops, you get hungry. That's why it's important to keep insulin levels low in the morning; it will keep your blood sugar levels constant and postpone hunger.

There's a phrase that goes "eating makes you hungry." The reason this is true is because eating is directly related to insulin levels. Once you start eating, the cycle of hormones begins to further stimulate hunger. If you've ever wondered why you wake up hungry after eating late in the evening, it's because insulin has been working through the night to transport the sugar out of your blood stream. Then, once you wake up, your body sees itself as needing to replenish its fuel, even though it really has plenty in storage. The same goes with eating in the morning—the sooner you eat, the more food you'll eat throughout the whole day.

You might be wondering if I'm dizzy or dazed by the time I finally sit down to eat. Not in the slightest. In fact, I have tons of energy all morning, and I even go right into my workouts. You see, eating well the day before fills up your body's gas tank and gives you the fuel and energy you need in the morning. Your body will use this stored fuel and burn it off first.

Another description of this way of eating is called intermittent fasting, which has proven in studies to have great health benefits. It has shown to lower insulin levels and increase production of fat-burning hormones, and it teaches your body how to go into your stored energy reserves, or fat, for fuel. This way of eating has also been linked to increased life span.

Think about breakfast as exactly what it is: breaking the fast. This can happen after seven hours of sleep or seven hours of activity—it's all about what you've eaten the day before to prepare your body. I recommend not going more than fifteen hours without food, which includes sleep time. The point is not to see how long you can go without eating; it's to set your body up to burn fat and function at its best. If you're still skeptical, just think about how waiting to break the fast will kick-start the fat-burning process by telling your body to literally burn fat—just imagine all that unwanted fat melting off you.

For your first meal of the day, I recommend you aim to eat protein or fat so you don't kick-start your hunger. You can certainly do exactly what I do, which is drink coffee only with full-fat cream—make sure it's regular half-and-half or heavy whipping cream, not fat-free or light. But I realize that not everyone is a coffee drinker, so if you need something a bit more substantial, try eggs, hard cheese, cottage cheese, peanut butter, nuts, or half of an avocado. The goal is to get just a little something in your stomach without spiking your insulin level. It goes without saying that you need to monitor the calories of whatever you eat, especially nuts and peanut butter. Whatever you do, do not eat high-carb foods first thing in the morning—this includes bagels, dry cereal, sugar, and muffins (pre-workout meals can be an exception; see page 78).

When it comes to evening, the kitchen is closed and I make sure I've had my last meal by six P.M. on most nights. That may seem really early, but I use it as a mental cutoff time to make sure I'm not eating during the last couple hours of the night. Like I said, I wake up at four A.M., but I still get eight hours of sleep, which means going to bed at eight P.M.

I like waking up feeling light—and not eating two hours before I fall asleep is the best way I can accomplish this. If I find myself eating after six P.M., it's rarely because I'm hungry; it's mostly because I'm bored. I am successful at keeping this cutoff time way more than 50 percent of the time, but not close to 100 percent. Obviously, if your bedtime is later, you can push back your eating cutoff time; just aim to quit eating two hours prior to when you go to bed. Most of the time, knowing how great

I feel in the morning if I make my cutoff time is enough to motivate me to stick with it. When you wake up in the morning feeling fresh and ready to face the day, instead of feeling full and tired, you'll thank me!

Social Smarts

When I think of what kind of curveballs can be thrown at you as you change your eating habits, at the top of the list are the well-meaning friends, family, and co-workers who invite us to lunch, dinner, parties, and potlucks. It seems everyone picks the least healthful dish they can find to share at a potluck—casseroles, over-the-top dips, cheap, tasteless cookies. Early on in my weight loss, I got to the point where I was practically offended by the pressure of having to be around foods of poor quality and outrageous quantity just so I could wish someone happy birthday.

I'm not trying to sound like a party pooper, but I think the party has moved far from focusing on the *people* at an event—the food is the star. Do people know how to do anything together besides eat? Here's what I do instead: I meet with friends for coffee or tea, or even better, I invite them over to my house where the good foods are, or we go for a walk at a park or in the neighborhood.

We've strayed so far from real connection of any sort. While you're reconnecting with your body, try to also reconnect with your friends, family, and neighbors, and rediscover the beauty of conversation and laughter. Believe it or not, you don't have to go out for a pizza or ice cream (not even frozen yogurt) to enjoy it.

And when it comes to having people over for food, if you've got goodies in the freezer, then you can be ready for almost anything within a very short period of time. I've pulled stuff out for company on more than one occasion, and when I make foods from scratch, it's so appreciated by my guests that they always leave asking for a recipe or two.

How to Eat Out

Once you've become accustomed to making your own foods with ingredients you've selected and portions you've created, you'll understand how pleasing it can be to eat meals at home that don't have a mysterious calorie count or ingredients. I used to get frustrated with having to eat out, but I discovered that I can be comfortable if I can get, at the very least, a decent salad and a freshly prepared piece of protein.

Consider the following uncommon common sense rules if you have to go to a restaurant, or even if it's your high-calorie day, but you still want to be smart:

- *Go to the highest-quality restaurant you can afford and skip the all-you-can-eat buffet.*
- *If you can't resist dessert, share a piece of cake with someone or even the whole table.*
- *Remember that you are paying for the meal—any ingredients you see on the menu can be made into what you want instead of what the restaurant staff has decided you might want. Order a hamburger patty to replace a processed piece of salty chicken on top of a salad, or you can order extra shredded cabbage or greens in your salads.*
- *Avoid cheese and cream sauces, and skip the bread or chips on the table before your meal.*
- *In general, always order a salad, but stay aware of all high-calorie additions like candied nuts, cheese, and salty meats like deli turkey or ham. Big dinner salads typically have all of these extras, so decide which ones you can live without—for me I leave off the nuts or cheese, or both.*
- *If none of the salad choices are good, then look for something on the menu that you would never cook at home so you can enjoy a bit of variety, but replace mashed potatoes or fries with extra veggies. You can also try sitting next to someone who doesn't overeat, or sharing a main course (fries and all) with your sweetie or a friend.*

Since you've stocked your house with fresh foods for your own meals, you can also always put out a tray of snacks that just happen to be delicious and healthful—you'll have plenty of options from which to choose. A plate with some good cheese, apple slices, olives, nuts, and fresh vegetables always goes over well with guests. Good food, real foods, live foods are the ingredients for a good life, and knowing how to use them will become first nature with practice.

Staying in the Zone

When you are in the zone, you eat right and you do your workouts as if they have always been a part of your life and they will never not be a part of your life. It's what you do, it's who you are, and it officially becomes your lifestyle—it changes from something you're doing into something you are.

I like to think of staying in the zone as similar to staying within your budget. Have you ever been late paying a bill, or maybe you just didn't have the money to pay it on time? Doesn't it make you feel bad? It's a monkey on your back, and sometimes you may wonder how you got yourself into that situation. Nothing feels better than being debt-free, except for maybe being fat-free. Think of the extra body weight you've been carrying as an unpaid debt to your body, and the only way to pay yourself back is to lose the weight. You've overdrawn the account by eating too much, and now it's time to pay up. During the week, you eat the foods your body needs and you stay within your caloric budget. At the end of the week, as long as you've stuck to your budget, you get the treat of losing weight and spending some extra calories.

Eating on the Move

It's important that you never leave your house without knowing what you are going to eat that day, or at the very least what your next meal is and/or where you are going to get it. Make no exceptions, and demand this from yourself and for yourself. If you don't plan to succeed, then you automatically plan to fail.

For years, I always put an apple in my bag before I left the house. Not a bag of apples, just one. I didn't have a plan for when I was going to eat it, but it was there when I didn't have time to eat a full meal, or when boredom hit and I felt like I needed to eat something. Lots of times I would eat an apple on my way home from work so I wouldn't arrive home starved and ready to overeat.

When it comes to longer trips away from home, I recommend packing as much of your own foods as possible. I rarely travel away from home for too long, and when I do it's almost always related to training and teaching at kettlebell certifications (lucky me—wherever I go there are kettlebells waiting for me!). When I do travel, I always pack at the very least a lunch to take with me. When I first started my diet, it was common for me to pack two to three days' worth of food on trips. I would take frozen soups on the plane with me or check them in my luggage and stock my hotel fridge with my own meals. This might

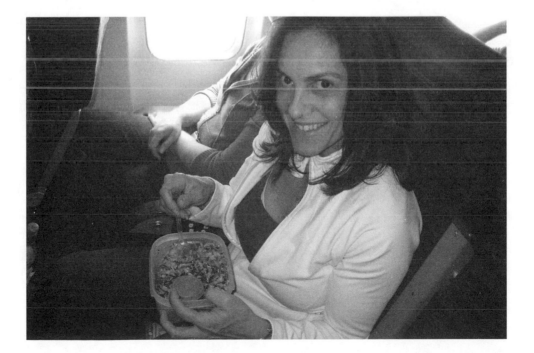

sound a bit extreme, but too often food in airports and on the road can be disappointing. Sometimes the only choices are complete junk food, and that can be extremely frustrating when you're motivated to stay on track.

At one point, I made an effort to relax about what and how much of my own foods I was bringing with me, but the choices were so blatantly salty, adding to the dehydration that comes along with travel, that I decided to go back to bringing better foods with me whenever possible. Once you've been in the zone, it always pulls you back to what is best for your body.

Here are some ideas for what to bring with you when you travel:

Prepared Cabbage Salads: I will carry one or two of these with me depending on the length of my trip. Put your dressing (see page 214 for my Asian Dressing recipe that's great on cabbage) on the bottom of the container and the shredded salad mix on top, and then mix it right before you eat it. Cabbage mixes can last for a long time, even close to a day without refrigeration. I add either pre-frozen, diced chicken so it lasts longer in transit until I eat it, or canned tuna. You can also find tuna in small, portable packets that you can open right before eating.

"Live" Trail Mix: I came up with this idea because I found myself eating too much trail mix from the bulk foods section at the grocery store—these are outrageously calorie-dense. Dried fruit and nuts add up fast and are not nearly as filling or satisfying when you take into account how small an actual serving size is. I'm always looking for ways to add fresh veggies to every meal because they are raw, crisp, and refreshing—they give this trail mix the "live" element. One of my absolute favorite snacks is peanut butter, raisins, and veggie sticks, so I decided to make this snack easy to eat by the handful by dicing up celery, carrots, and broccoli stalks into the size of nuts. I add raisins and peanuts to this, and then I have "live" trail mix! I love this snack, and it's perfect to have on a plane flight that lasts for hours. You can even use the airline-provided peanuts in the little packets they give you.

Fresh Fruit: Fruits like apples and grapes are easy to carry with you. If you bring grapes, pack no more than ⅓ pound, which is about 100 calories. I also will add grapes into my salad, so those do double duty acting as a snack and a salad topper.

Cheeses: I'm not talking about processed slices of American, but good quality pieces of cheeses like Manchego, smoked Gouda, or Dubliner. Good cheeses taste better at room temperature, and they taste great with a few grapes or a slice of an apple. You can also pick up Mini Babybels, which are pre-wrapped, have about 70 calories apiece, and will last awhile in your bag.

Nuts and Prunes: If I throw these in a little resealable bag, they'll last an entire trip, but I have to snack on them cautiously—it's far too easy to overdo it with this type of snack. You can have five prunes or fifteen almonds for around 100 calories.

You can also pack some crackers or a peanut butter sandwich made with one slice of bread. Just be careful with the more calorie-dense foods, as the boredom of travel can lure you into eating even when you're not hungry.

You can often find a lot of these on the road when you're traveling—there are grocery stores just about everywhere. Personally, I have my favorite brands, and it takes so little time to throw together while still at home, I prefer to pack everything with me.

Falling in Love with Real Foods

Creating the habits and skills that allow you to become fast and efficient in food preparation is only part of your eating habit makeover. Reacquainting your taste buds with real foods—the foods we naturally crave but have lost touch with—is an essential part of the process as well. We are our bodies; they are the physical representation of ourselves, and they determine our experience of every moment. Your body can either distract you from the full experience you are meant to have, or it can enhance and empower it. The quality of the building blocks, or the food you put into your body, directly determines the quality of every bit of you—from your cells to your organs to your skin, heart, and brain—isn't it time you built the body you've always dreamed of?

· ·

Tracy's Food Rule #9: You Can Soften the Blow

One of the most common complaints people make when they start to eat real foods is how bland they taste. I have news for you—if your diet consists mostly of processed foods, especially fast foods, then you have been assaulting and deceiving your taste buds for too long. The food industry pumps processed foods full of salt, sugars, and fat to keep us coming back for more. I know how alluring it can be—I was under the powerful spell of these foods for years. The problem is, the satisfaction ends in your mouth; your body is left dealing with the trash that remains.

If you think healthful foods taste bad, then there are ways of weaning yourself off of over-flavored foods by diluting them with fresh choices. Diluting over-flavored foods with healthier ingredients is one of my favorite ways of getting the taste of calorie-dense convenience foods without doing all the damage. For instance, if you love something like McDonald's cheeseburgers (as I did), instead of ordering three (as I would), buy one without the cheese (330 calories with cheese, 250 without), and cut it into a dozen bites, bun and all. Then, toss it with a salad made of nutritious greens and a dressing made with 1 tablespoon mayo, 1 tablespoon ketchup, and 2 tablespoons plain yogurt. By doing this, you double the volume of the hamburger, or junk food of your choice, while cutting the calories by two thirds.

You can also try this with sushi: cut each piece into quarters, toss it with some shredded Chinese cabbage, a little extra rice vinegar, soy sauce, 1–2 teaspoons of sesame oil, and you triple the volume of your meal while only adding a few calories.

I also used to use this same strategy when making healthful but less calorie-conscious meals for my family. I would take 2 cups of a basic vegetable soup I had made and add to it whatever main course I had cooked—lasagna, spaghetti, risotto, tacos—just about anything tastes good in a vegetable soup. The flavors enrich the soup, and you never feel that you've missed out on anything. The funny part is, as I started to eat better, my family began gravitating toward my foods.

• •

12 Recipes for Real Life

As you read through many of these recipes, you'll notice how basic a lot of them are (I'm trying to get you to cook, not become a chef). I was tempted to go all out and list many more choices, but you don't need more choices, you need fewer. I suggest reading through this chapter and selecting one or two of the recipes to start with.

Once you've picked a couple, try to make them over and over again until you start to feel comfortable preparing and making them. This way, you'll build your confidence and improve your cooking skills as you give yourself a nice foundation on which to build. The more often you repeat a recipe, the more likely you will keep the necessary ingredients on hand, and you'll find it makes your weekly shopping easier.

Onion Recipes

Before you scan right over these because you think you don't like onions, I'd like to make a quick request: give onions a chance! Not only do they provide an amazing base flavor to foods, they also have some surprising health benefits. Onions have the same anti-inflammatory properties of garlic, and they've been shown to help reduce the risk of certain types of cancer. They've also been proven to help prevent blood clotting and increase bone density. My personal mantra is "chop an onion a day"— following this simple rule will help you get in the habit of making your own fresh and flavorful foods.

Fresh Salsa

Makes: 2 servings

Salsa counts as 0 calories on the Swing Diet, and once you taste this version, you might find yourself wanting to put it on everything. When you get into the habit of making fresh salsa, you'll wonder why you ever bought it premade. Pretty soon all your friends will be asking you to bring your salsa to parties. Try using just salsa as a condiment instead of other high-calorie options. You can also add it to the Guacamole Smoothie (see page 204) for some extra flavor or use it as a dip for Salad on a Stick (see page 223).

> ½ white onion, chopped
> 2 large tomatoes, diced
> 1 fresh jalapeño pepper, finely diced
> ½ bunch cilantro, chopped
> 1–2 tablespoons fresh lime juice
> 1 garlic clove, crushed
> Salt

Mix all ingredients together in a bowl. Start with a pinch of salt and add more until it brings out the flavors.

Caramelized Onion Soup

Makes: 4 servings

You will be slicing, not dicing, onions for this recipe. To cut onions to be caramelized, cut in half from stem to root, and then place the flat side down and cut off both the stem and root. From there, cut into thin slices with the knife running from stem to root.

6–8 medium yellow onions, sliced (these will cook down quite a bit)

2 tablespoons olive oil (or 1 tablespoon butter, 1 tablespoon olive oil)

Red pepper flakes (optional)

Salt

4–6 cups chicken stock

To make caramelized onions: Heat large skillet on medium high. Add olive oil or mixture to the hot pan; add onions, a good pinch each of salt and red pepper flakes, and stir to coat. Cook until onions start to soften, and reduce heat to medium. Continue to cook another 25–30 minutes, turning every 5–8 minutes. If the bottom of the pan starts to get dark and dry, add a little water (¼ cup) to loosen and clean up all of the brown bits on the bottom of the pan (this is called deglazing the pan).

To make soup: Transfer onions to a larger stockpot, if needed. Add chicken stock and cook until heated through. You can also make this a heartier main dish by adding 2–4 ounces of cooked Italian sausage or roasted chicken, and topping with a handful of croutons or an ounce of shredded Swiss or Parmesan cheese.

Onion Pepper Sauce and Pasta

Makes: 4 servings

4 tablespoons olive oil (or 2 tablespoons butter, 2 tablespoons olive oil)

6–8 medium yellow onions, sliced

2–4 red bell peppers, thinly sliced

2 tablespoons balsamic vinegar

½ package (8 ounces) spaghetti noodles, cooked

2 ounces grated Parmesan cheese

Heat large skillet on medium high. Add olive oil or mixture to the hot pan; add onions and bell peppers, and stir to coat. Cook until onions and peppers start to soften, and reduce heat to medium. Continue to cook another 25–30 minutes, turning every 5–8 minutes. When the onions and peppers are just about finished, deglaze the pan with balsamic vinegar, toss with cooked spaghetti noodles, and top with cheese. Use the leftover pasta water to thin out the sauce, if needed.

You can also make this into a hearty soup by adding 1–2 cups of hot chicken stock, 2–4 ounces of protein, and a handful of spinach, which will wilt in the soup.

202

Perfect Pasta Noodles

How to cook dry pasta: I never use an entire one-pound box of dry pasta because it's so high in calories. If you use double the vegetables in the sauce, you won't miss the extra noodles. Cook noodles according to package directions, but what you won't find there is how much salt to add. I learned in Tuscany, Italy, that pasta water is traditionally seasoned with two tablespoons of salt. I now add this much salt to 6–8 quarts of pasta water, and since adopting this secret, my family loves my pasta dishes. Before draining your pasta, get in the habit of saving at least ½ cup of the pasta water to thin your sauce if needed.

Smoothies

Before I decided to lose weight, I would frequent Jamba Juice, and even though I wasn't trying to eat fewer calories at the time, I often got one of the two smoothies they offered with real yogurt instead of frozen yogurt. When it was time for me to design my own eating guidelines, I knew I could make a more nutritious and better-quality smoothie by using my favorite brand of yogurt and fresh ingredients. And I knew I could make it for much cheaper than five dollars a pop.

I never recommend using non-fat dairy products because the calorie difference isn't that significant and low-fat or full-fat dairy options are much more satisfying. Also, try to use fresh seasonal fruits when possible, and when they're ripe, freeze extras to save for later. To freeze fruits, rinse them off in cold water (dice any fruit larger than berries), line them up on a sheet of wax paper so they're not touching, and then place them in the freezer for an hour or so. Once they're solid enough so they won't stick together, put them in an airtight container and freeze for later use.

Plain Yogurt Smoothie

Makes: 1 serving

> 8 ounces plain yogurt
>
> 2 tablespoons honey (or sugar, maple syrup, or sweetener of your choice)
>
> 1 cup fresh or frozen strawberries (or amount of fruit of your choice that equals 100 calories)
>
> ½ cup ice
>
> ½ cup water
>
> 2 tablespoons psyllium fiber (optional)

Blend all items together until you've achieved desired consistency.

Vanilla Yogurt Smoothie

Makes: 1 serving

> 8 ounces vanilla yogurt
>
> ¾–1 cup fresh or frozen fruit
>
> ½ cup ice
>
> ½ cup water
>
> 2 tablespoons psyllium fiber (optional)

Blend all items together until you've achieved desired consistency. You can use any flavor of yogurt you'd like, but be sure to keep an eye on the calories.

Cottage Cheese Smoothies

Recently I started to make my smoothies with cottage cheese instead of yogurt because it has more protein and it gives them a slightly richer flavor and thicker consistency. Before you think it sounds strange, consider how delicious a cheesecake is with cottage cheese or ricotta. A cottage cheese smoothie can be sweet or savory, like my Guacamole Smoothie. If your diet is too high in salty foods already, watch the sodium in cottage cheese because it's more than what you will get in yogurt.

◗ Roasted Butternut Squash Smoothie

Makes: 1 serving

Once roasted, winter squashes can be cut into pre-portioned pieces and then refrigerated or frozen for future soups and smoothies. Winter squashes are more starch based and count as a carb serving, like a potato. Never have more than one starchy carb vegetable portion per day.

> ¾ cup cottage cheese
>
> 1–2 tablespoons sugar (or brown sugar, honey, or maple syrup)
>
> ½–1 cup roasted butternut squash
>
> ½ cup ice
>
> ½ cup water
>
> A handful of spinach (optional, but why not?)

Cut 1 butternut squash in half and place face up on a roasting sheet in a 400°F oven. Cook until soft, when a fork easily pierces flesh. Depending on the size, this should take about 30–45 minutes. Seeding it is much easier after it's cooked (and more convenient too!). Cool, then cut up for use in your smoothie or save for later.

To make smoothie: Remove skin from butternut squash. Add 1 cup of squash to blender and blend with remaining ingredients until you've achieved desired consistency.

◗ Guacamole Smoothie

Makes: 1 serving

Of course, you have to take into consideration that avocado is counted as fat nutritionally, so I never use more than ⅓ of a medium avocado. And in this case, I use low-fat cottage cheese because of the fat in the avocado.

> ¾ cup low-fat cottage cheese
>
> ⅓ medium avocado
>
> ½–¾ cup Fresh Salsa (see page 200)
>
> 1 lime, juiced
>
> 2 teaspoons sugar (or to taste, up to an additional teaspoon)
>
> Salt
>
> ½ cup ice
>
> ½ cup water
>
> A handful of spinach or fresh cilantro

Blend all items together until you've achieved desired consistency. You can also add black pepper or a bit of cayenne pepper if you like a spicy flavor.

Oatmeal and Other Hot Cereals

I love oatmeal because it reminds me of my childhood. I remember having it for breakfast every morning before going out to wait for the school bus. Thanks to those memories, I still like my oatmeal with plain old white sugar and milk.

I like thick, old-fashioned oats, which are the kind that take about five minutes to cook. You can have any other hot cereal like Cream of Wheat, multigrain, or even grits—whatever makes you happy. I'm not going to argue about nutritional differences as long as you stay within the serving size. I always start with two cups of water to make sure I get a healthy portion without adding more calories.

Oatmeal or other hot cereals are easy to make ahead of time even for the whole week if you don't mind reheated or microwaved foods. It does get thick, but for me the pros outweigh the cons.

Don't be afraid of a little creativity when you eat oatmeal. When I make mine sweet, it's kind of like dessert, so I will have it for dinner—it makes me feel like I've ended my day with dessert, which is always nice. Since it's a carb meal, it also helps me sleep better.

Oatmeal

Makes: 1 serving

> 2 cups water
> ½ cup old-fashioned oats
> Salt

Cook oatmeal according to package directions. There are plenty of options for adding flavor:

- Sweetener of your choice: As long as you count the calories, you can use up to 2 tablespoons, or about 90 calories, of a sweetener.
- Dried fruit: Dried raisins, blueberries, or cranberries can take the place of all or some of the sweetener. Or you can use fresh fruit.
- Milk, yogurt, or cottage cheese: Add ¼–½ cup of one of these choices. Try them all— you might find a new favorite way to have oatmeal.
- Zero-calorie spices: Try cinnamon, pumpkin pie spice, or vanilla extract for some extra "free" flavor.
- Nuts: Sliced almonds, walnuts, or pecans are great in oatmeal, but watch the calories.
- Savory option: Add 1 ounce of crumbled feta cheese, or some other hard cheese, and a generous grind of black pepper.

Meat Proteins

My favorite way to get protein is to prepare large portions of meats ahead of time and then add them to soups or salads during the week to make them heartier and more flavorful. Of course, you can always eat meat separately as more of an entrée, but be sure to watch your portions. When preparing meats, it's best to bring them out of the refrigerator at least 30 minutes before cooking, if possible. Room temperature meats cook more evenly and don't dry out as easily.

Poached Chicken Breast

Makes: 2 servings

Roasting a whole chicken is ideal, but simply poaching some chicken breasts is a good alternative that takes less time and energy. Chicken breasts are most commonly sold in halves. The breast is cut down the center sternum, and the result is two halves, even though most people think they're getting a whole breast.

> 4 cups chicken broth
> 2 boneless chicken breast halves

Bring chicken broth to a rolling boil and slide chicken breasts into boiling liquid. Turn off the heat and cover pot with a tight-fitting lid. Leave covered for 20 minutes—do not lift cover until 20 minutes has passed, as you will remove some of the heat. To check doneness, insert a meat thermometer into chicken; a fully cooked chicken breast will have an internal temperature of 165°F.

Pan-Roasted Pork Tenderloin with Chinese Marinade

Makes: 8 servings

I always cook two tenderloins at the same time. No extra effort is needed, and besides, when I make this recipe I've got to race the rest of my family to it before it disappears. If you have leftovers, they will keep up to four days in the refrigerator.

⅓ cup soy sauce

¼ cup vinegar

2 teaspoons five-spice

3 tablespoon olive oil (1 tablespoon reserved for browning)

2 teaspoons Chinese hot mustard, or hot sauce and yellow mustard

1–2 garlic cloves, crushed

2 pork tenderloins with silverskin removed (have the butcher do this for you)

Mix together first six ingredients and pour into a resealable bag or bowl. Add pork tenderloins to the marinade, seal tightly, and place in refrigerator for 2–6 hours.

To make tenderloins: Preheat oven to 400°F. Remove meat from marinade and place in an ovenproof skillet. On the stovetop, brown all sides of the tenderloins in reserved oil, and then transfer to oven. Check temperature with an instant-read thermometer after 15 minutes, and then every 5–10 minutes until internal temperature reaches 155–160°F. Total cooking time should be around 20 minutes but will vary based on your oven. Remove from oven and tent with foil. Let stand 15 minutes.

Tenting Meats

Once you take meat out of the oven or off the grill, it's often best to tent it to make sure it stays warm, but it's also important to make sure it doesn't overcook. Remove meat from heat source, and then place on a cutting board. To tent, fold a big piece of aluminum foil over meat and form it into a loose tent that's draped about one to two inches above the meat. Pinch the edges of the foil onto your cutting board so the tent stays in place. The resting time will vary based on the type of meat you've prepared, but typically it's about 10-15 minutes.

Butterflied Leg of Lamb with Spice Rub

Makes: 8–10 servings

> 2 tablespoons chopped fresh rosemary
> 1 tablespoon black pepper
> 2–4 garlic cloves, minced
> 2 tablespoons sugar
> ¼ cup salt
> 1 boneless leg of lamb (around 4 pounds)

Mix together first five ingredients. Rub whole leg of lamb with mixture and refrigerate 4–6 hours or overnight.

To make lamb: Take meat out of fridge at least 30 minutes before cooking. Rinse spice mixture off and towel dry. Preheat outdoor grill or, if broiling, broiler and broiler pan. Cook lamb approximately 25–30 minutes, turning every 6–8 minutes. Check temperature in the thickest part of meat and remove at 130°F for medium rare. Tent with foil and let stand 15 minutes before slicing.

Skirt Steak with Bourbon Marinade

Makes: 6 servings

> 2 tablespoons olive oil
> 2 tablespoons mustard (any kind is fine)
> ¼ cup bourbon whiskey
> ¼ cup soy sauce
> 2 tablespoons red wine, or cider vinegar
> 2 tablespoons brown sugar
> 1 tablespoon salt, or garlic salt
> 2 teaspoons freshly ground black pepper
> 2 skirt steaks (about 2–3 pounds)

Mix together all ingredients except for steak and pour into a resealable bag or bowl. Add skirt steaks to mix, seal tightly, and place in refrigerator for 2–4 hours or overnight.

To make steaks: Take steaks out of fridge about 30 minutes before cooking. Remove meat from marinade and dry off with paper towels. Using a sharp knife, cut big crosshatches on both sides of the steaks. Broil or grill for 4–5 minutes on each side. Let rest for 10–15 minutes and cut across the grain into thin slices.

Salads

Before I turned thirty-four—when I learned to cook—I had never bought a head of cabbage or even knew what one looked like. In fact, I had never bought a lot of the ingredients in these recipes before I learned how to cook. I couldn't identify most fresh vegetables by sight, much less fresh herbs. What I finally discovered is that there are some incredible flavors and textures out there to be experienced that can completely change your definition of "salad." I hope you'll be open and adventurous when it comes to trying new vegetables.

Some of the best salads are made from vegetables that people tradition-ally only eat cooked. For example, cauliflower, asparagus, and beets are all delicious raw. Raw veggie salads are perfect for a traveling lunch because they stay crisp longer without refrigeration and taste better at room temp.

· ·

Smart Salad Prep

To help with food preparation for salads (and other recipes as well), I recommend investing in a mandoline or V-slicer if you don't have a food processor with a slicing blade. I like the one made by OXO—it is a must for pre-shredding jobs.

You can also use a basic vegetable peeler to prepare some vegetables. I often use one to make carrot ribbons for my salads. Just do a quick swipe to peel the skin off, and then keep peeling and let the long strips drop into your salad mix. This works to shred cabbage too, if you're only making one serving.

These days most grocery stores carry packages of pre-shredded cabbage and broccoli in addition to all kinds of prepackaged salad greens and prepped vegetables, so you can always go that route if you have to. Either way, no excuses!

· ·

Basic Cabbage Salad Mix

Makes: 3–4 servings

This is a perfect everyday salad mix that will serve as a base salad to most of the other salad recipes you'll find here. I prefer cabbage as the main ingredient in this salad because it's flavorful and has a fantastic crunch to it. I'll make this mix and pre-portion into containers to keep in the refrigerator. Then, I'll make single-serving salads from those portions all week—the salad stays fresh and crisp as long as you don't pre-dress it. Tasty, simple, and best of all, extremely quick!

> 1 head green cabbage, shredded
> ½ head red cabbage, shredded
> 2 carrots, shredded
> 1 bunch green onions, thinly sliced
> 1–2 fresh jalapeños, diced small
> Cilantro or any fresh herb of your choice (optional)

Add all ingredients to a large bowl and toss.

A Tempting Salad

This is the one of my most requested recipes. It's a favorite of mine, and it's sure to become a favorite of yours. Don't be surprised when your co-workers walk by and, once they get a whiff of your salad, ask: "Did you make that? It smells delicious!"

Chicken Curry Coleslaw with Curry Dressing

Makes: 1 large serving (salad); 6 servings (dressing)

> 3–4 cups loosely packed Basic Cabbage Salad Mix
> 2–4 ounces chicken breast, diced
> ¼ cup golden raisins, or 3–4 ounces grapes, halved (optional)

> For dressing:
> 8 ounces plain low-fat yogurt
> 4 ounces mayonnaise
> 2 tablespoons lemon juice

2 tablespoons cider vinegar

2 tablespoons sugar (or honey)

1–2 tablespoons curry powder

2–4 garlic cloves, crushed

1 teaspoon salt

Whisk together all dressing ingredients. Pour ¼–⅓ cup over cabbage mixture and toss, coating the vegetables and chicken. Store unused dressing in refrigerator; it keeps for at least one week.

Turkey Waldorf Coleslaw with Blue Cheese Dressing

Makes: 1 large serving (salad); 6 servings (dressing)

3–4 cups loosely packed Basic Cabbage Salad Mix

1 stalk celery, thinly sliced

½–1 apple, diced (or 3–4 ounces grapes, or ¼ cup dried cranberries)

2–4 ounces turkey breast, diced

For dressing:

8 ounces low-fat yogurt or buttermilk

2 ounces mayonnaise

3 ounces blue cheese

1 garlic clove, crushed

Worcestershire sauce, to taste

Whisk together all dressing ingredients. Add ¼–⅓ cup dressing to salad mixture and toss to coat. Store unused dressing in refrigerator; it keeps for at least one week.

Broccoli Crunch Salad with Tuna

Makes: 1 large serving

Did you know that a whole can of tuna is only around 150 calories? I think a big mistake dieters make (I know I've made this mistake more than once) is to try to cut calories too low. What happens then is you get so hungry, you give in to something you didn't even want in the first place. So remember—you have to eat to lose weight.

1 can tuna packed in water, drained

1 tablespoon mayonnaise

1–2 cups loosely packed Basic Cabbage Salad Mix

½–¾ cup chopped broccoli

1 serving grapes (4 ounces); or 1 small apple, diced; or 1 ounce golden raisins
or dried cranberries

2 tablespoons low-calorie dressing (not to exceed 40 calories per tablespoon)

In a bowl, mix tuna with mayonnaise. Then add to cabbage salad mix and distribute throughout. I usually add my favorite low-calorie Asian peanut dressing for a bit of extra flavor.

Raw Cauliflower Salad with Black Beans, Corn, and Tomato

Makes: 4 large servings

This salad is great with fancy-shmancy baby tomatoes from the farmers' market. If you can make it with seasonal, fresh roasted corn, it will be even tastier. This is when a food processor, mandolin, or V-slicer will come in handy to finely slice cauliflower.

1 head of cauliflower, sliced super fine

1–2 ears of fresh corn, roasted and cut from cob

½ cup black beans

1 basket baby tomatoes, or 1 cup diced red tomato

4 tablespoons white wine vinegar

Squeeze of lemon juice

2 tablespoons olive oil

Salt and pepper, to taste

1–2 teaspoons sugar, if needed

Mix cauliflower, corn, beans, and tomatoes together in a large bowl. Add vinegar, lemon juice, and olive oil, and toss salad. Sprinkle with salt and pepper, and take a sample bite; add sugar as needed to bring out corn and tomato flavors.

Asparagus, Red Onion, and Pecorino Salad

Makes: 2 servings

This is a favorite salad I learned from Chef Ann Burrell on her show *Secrets of a Restaurant Chef*. I've modified it to fit better into the parameters of my diet. This salad is best in spring when asparagus is in season and you can find the really thin and tender bunches.

2 bunches tender asparagus, raw and thinly sliced

½ red onion, finely diced

⅓ cup pecorino Romano cheese, grated

2–4 tablespoons red wine vinegar (can add more as needed)

2 tablespoons olive oil

Salt and pepper, to taste

Toss all ingredients together; cover and place in refrigerator at least 2 hours to let the flavors blend.

- -

Asparagus, Mushroom, and Pecorino Salad

Here's another great-tasting twist on this simple recipe: substitute sherry vinegar for the red wine vinegar, diced shallot for the red onion, and add sliced mushrooms. Delicious!

- -

Red and Gold Raw Beet Salad

Makes: 2 servings

Keep the two beet colors separate until just before you eat it, or you will end up with only red beet salad. Once you start to incorporate fresh vegetables as the base of your meals, you'll begin to appreciate the beautiful colors of natural foods—they always say your plate should look like a rainbow. This salad is gorgeous to look at and delicious to eat. The grating disk on your food processor makes quick work of this, but I use a simple box cheese grater—just watch your fingers.

1 medium red beet, grated

1 medium golden beet, grated

1 carrot, grated

2–3 green onions, thinly sliced

½ bunch of the beet greens, cut into thin ribbons

1 fresh jalapeño, finely diced (optional)

2 tablespoons chopped cilantro (optional)

¾ cup fresh pineapple chunks, or 4–6 chopped dates (my favorite sweet add-ins)

Separate beet stems from the leaves, and wash and dry beet greens. To prep the greens, stack the leaves one on top of the other lengthwise and cut across the width into thin ribbons. Add all ingredients to a large bowl and toss. Drizzle with ¼ cup Asian Dressing (see below) and mix thoroughly. I like to add grilled prawns, chicken, or Pan-Roasted Pork Tenderloin with Chinese Marinade (see page 207) to this salad.

Asian Dressing

Makes: 4 servings

This dressing is oil-based and should be measured to ensure you don't use too much. It can be made in the food processor, and it's a favorite of mine to dress my Red and Gold Raw Beet Salad (see above). It's also a great addition to any slaw made with Chinese (Napa) cabbage or any type of radish.

> 2 garlic cloves, minced
> 1 tablespoon grated ginger
> ¼ cup rice wine vinegar
> 1–2 tablespoons soy sauce
> 2 tablespoons sugar or honey
> 1 teaspoon Sriracha or Tabasco, if you want it spicy
> ¼ cup peanut oil (or whatever oil you prefer)
> 2 teaspoons toasted sesame oil

Mix garlic, ginger, vinegar, soy sauce, sugar, and hot sauce together. Drizzle in peanut oil and sesame oil; whisk together. This dressing can be stored in the refrigerator one week. As a general rule, any dressing made with fresh ingredients like garlic or onion will last about one week.

Basic Caesar Salad

Makes: 1 large serving (salad); 6 servings (dressing)

As good as a Basic Caesar Salad is, throwing in some leftover grilled or roasted veggies makes it amazing. I will gladly pass on the croutons and Parmesan cheese in trade for roasted or grilled veggies.

4 cups chopped romaine lettuce, loosely packed

2–4 ounces chicken or turkey breast, diced

For dressing:

8 ounces plain yogurt

4 ounces mayonnaise

2–4 tablespoons lemon juice

2–4 cloves garlic, crushed

Salt and pepper, to taste

4 anchovy fillets, finely chopped, or 2 tablespoons anchovy paste

Mix lettuce and chicken in a bowl. Combine all dressing ingredients together in a separate bowl and whisk until it has a smooth consistency. Pour ¼–⅓ cup over salad mixture and toss, coating the vegetables and chicken. Store unused dressing in refrigerator; it keeps for at least one week. If you are using anchovy filets, add them to the top of the salad.

· ·

Caesar Options

You can find anchovy paste in the Italian food section of most stores. Before you think that you don't like anchovy, try it first. There's so little anchovy in this dressing, it's added mostly for its saltiness and only has a hint of fish flavor. If you don't like it after you try it, you can use capers or caper paste (you will find it next to the anchovy paste), or finely chopped kalamata olives.

· ·

The Best-Tasting Vegetables You've Ever Had

I'm probably the only woman in America who doesn't have a husband who grills. And because of that, I don't own a grill, which is pretty outrageous when you live in California. Luckily, I have a stovetop grill, which can make just as tasty vegetables. If you don't have either, I suggest picking up a basic grill pan. Grilling couldn't get any easier, and when you cook vegetables this way, they're crispy and caramelized and the taste is out of this world. The only thing you should be careful about is the amount of olive oil you use on your veggies before grilling.

I usually prep my vegetables and put them all in a large stainless mixing bowl. To this I will add a generous amount of salt and a good pinch or two of red pepper flakes. I then measure 2 tablespoons olive oil and drizzle it in a thin stream over and around the veggies as well as close to the inside rim of the bowl. The oil drizzles down the sides of the bowl and begins to gently coat the vegetables. I mix, stir, and massage them with the oil using my hands.

Remember to preheat your grill—you should always hear a sizzle when you place your veggies down. Sliced zucchini, bell peppers, onion, asparagus, and corn can take as little as a few minutes on each side. To roast corn, you can place whole shucked cobs on the gas flame (without any oil or other added fat) on your stove top and turn every few minutes, cooking and turning until some of the kernels blacken. Let cool and cut kernels away from cob. You can do the same on an outdoor grill.

Don't be afraid of getting a little creative—vegetables like chard, lettuce, and cabbage taste great grilled. For lettuce and cabbage, cut heads in half or quarters, leaving the core intact (this is what holds it together). For kale, you can just cut or tear large leaves into two to three pieces. Drizzle them with a bit of olive oil, salt, and stick them right on a hot grill or grill pan for a few minutes on each side. Chop when cool enough to handle.

Grilled Vegetable and Quinoa Salad

Makes: 4 servings

This salad is so simple and quick. I'll give you my favorite combination of veggies, but you can make your own substitutions as you discover what vegetables you like roasted or on the grill. Quinoa can be replaced with brown rice, lentils, or beans, but just be sure to load up on the veggies and not the grains and legumes.

2 cups cooked quinoa

1–2 ears of corn, grilled or roasted, kernels cut from the cob

2 small green and yellow zucchini squash, sliced ¼ inch lengthwise for grilling, then diced large for salad

1 6-ounce package baby salad greens or baby spinach

2 tomatoes, diced (or 1 basket baby tomatoes, halved)

1 ounce crumbled feta cheese

1–2 tablespoons olive oil

1–2 lemons, juiced

Salt and pepper, to taste

Make quinoa according to package directions and keep warm while you prepare the other veggies for the salad. Grill or roast corn and squash, and add with the tomatoes to salad greens. The oil on the grilled veggies will help wilt the baby greens and/or spinach. Add quinoa, crumble cheese over top, and drizzle with olive oil—you won't need much more because there's oil on the vegetables (be sure that between the oil in the veggies and the oil drizzled in, you use no more than two tablespoons of olive oil). Add lemon juice and salt and pepper.

Substitutes or Additions:
- Cucumber
- Radish, thinly sliced
- Grilled or roasted red bell pepper
- Asparagus
- Grilled scallions, cut into 1-inch pieces
- Blanched green beans
- Queso fresco or cotija cheese (instead of feta)

A Better Grain

Quinoa contains more protein than any other grain; an average of just over 16 percent, with some varieties having more than 20 percent protein. Rice is only 7.5 percent protein, and wheat is 14 percent. Quinoa is also unique in that it's what's known as a complete protein, which means it contains all of the essential amino acids. Plus, it's gluten-free.

Soups and Stews

The difference between soup and stew is that soups tend to have more broth and stews tend to have more meat and vegetables, making them a bit heartier. Most soups and stews begin with a combination of onion, celery, and carrot, otherwise known as mirepoix (see page 180 for more on this French term). Then you add in garlic and spices, and this creates the first layer of flavor of just about every soup or stew recipe, no matter the country of origin. This is why it's so important to know how to prep vegetables—they'll be the base of all your most delicious meals.

A chili, on the other hand, is made with . . . well, chilies. If you add a jalapeño pepper, a pasilla pepper, or a red bell pepper to a vegetable soup base and toss in some chili powder, you have chili. Of course, you can make it heartier and better tasting by adding tomatoes, meat, beans, and more spices. I'm not trying to define a traditional chili—for our purposes, the only requirement is that it tastes good and spicy, and that it's nutritious (which will come naturally since you're using real ingredients).

Basic Veggie Soup

Makes: 4 servings

> ½ head cabbage, sliced into ½-inch ribbons
> 1 small onion, finely diced
> 2 carrots, small dice
> 2–3 celery stalks, medium dice
> ½ bunch Tuscan kale, leaves separated, small dice (stems are optional)
> 1–2 garlic cloves, chopped or crushed
> 2 cups chicken stock (I use homemade)
> Salt and pepper, to taste

Sauté onion, carrot, celery, and kale stems (if using them) in olive oil for 5 minutes. Add cabbage and stir to coat with oil; cook for another 5 minutes. When the vegetables begin to caramelize, add the garlic. Continue cooking for 1 minute, and then add stock. Deglaze the bottom of the pan (with stock), add in chopped kale leaves, and bring to a boil. Reduce heat to low and partially cover for 15 min.

Make it Southwest: Add 1 tablespoon of oregano and 1 tablespoon ground cumin at the same time you add the garlic. When soup is done, add 2–4 ounces of cooked chicken or pork, and ½ cup black beans and/or corn per serving. Finish with a dollop of yogurt, sour cream, or cheese.

Make it Italian: Add 1 tablespoon oregano and 1 teaspoon dried rosemary, or 1 tablespoon Italian seasoning at the same time you add the garlic. Add 1 small can diced tomatoes and 1–2 small zucchini, diced, along with stock. When soup is finished, add 2–4 ounces of cooked Italian sausage or chicken. You can also add ½ cup of cooked white beans per serving.

Make it Indian: Add 2 teaspoons garam masala or curry powder at the same time as the garlic. Add 1 can light coconut milk and 1 small can tomatoes when you add stock. If using uncooked lentils, add two cups additional stock or water and 1 cup green or red lentils, rinsed; cook for an additional 25 minutes. Add chopped cauliflower florets in the last 15 minutes of cooking time. When soup is done, add 2–4 ounces of cooked lamb, chicken, or turkey. Watch the coconut milk, as even the light version can be high in calories.

Red Chili

Makes: 6 servings

Don't be intimidated by the long list of ingredients you see here. This chili is amazing, and it only gets better as the flavors meld together over a couple days. It also freezes and thaws out for a perfect quick lunch or dinner. Top with freshly chopped onions or a tablespoon of grated cheese.

    1 pound ground beef, pork, turkey, chicken, or a combination of any of these
    1–2 tablespoons olive oil
    1 onion, diced
    2 stalks celery, diced
    2 carrots, diced
    1 red bell pepper, small dice
    2–4 jalapeño peppers, small dice
    1–2 garlic cloves, crushed
    2 tablespoons chili powder or chipotle powder (chipotle powder has a
        smoky flavor)
    1 tablespoon ground cumin

1 tablespoon dried oregano

1 teaspoon each of dried thyme and fennel (only if using pork or poultry)

1–2 canned chipotle peppers (individual peppers, not 1–2 cans; these will be removed before serving)

1 small can diced tomatoes, including liquid

2–4 tablespoons tomato paste

1 can of cooked beans (black, red, or pinto)

4 cups chicken stock

Salt and pepper, to taste

In a deep skillet, brown meat(s). Then remove from pan, drain fat, and set aside. In the same pan, heat olive oil. When hot, add onion, celery, carrots, red bell pepper, and jalapeño peppers; sauté for 5–6 minutes or until soft. Add garlic and cook for 1 minute. Add dry spices and chipotle peppers, and once fragrant (another 1–2 minutes), stir in diced tomatoes, tomato paste, cooked beans, and chicken stock. Bring to a boil, reduce heat, and simmer 15–20 minutes.

Sprinkle with salt and pepper. Remove 2 cups of chili and puree in a blender or food processor (this will thicken the chili); return to pot. Add cooked ground meat and reheat, if necessary.

Pureed Veggie Soups

Makes: 4 servings

I'm going to give you the easiest of the easy methods for making pureed soups, and then a method that's just slightly more time consuming.

4–6 cups veggies, cut into ½–1-inch pieces (summer squash, zucchini, yellow squash, pattypans, crookneck, broccoli, cauliflower, tomato, butternut squash)

2–4 cups chicken stock

Salt and pepper, to taste

Put cut vegetables into a large pot with enough chicken stock to barely cover, and cook until vegetables are tender; check with a fork after about 10 minutes. Let veggies cool until you can safely add them to a blender. Blend and add more stock until you reach the desired consistency. Season with salt and pepper.

To make when you have more time: In a stockpot, sauté mirepoix (see page 180) in 1 tablespoon olive oil until onion is translucent. Add prepped vegetables and chicken stock to cover. Proceed with remaining steps of previous recipe. This method doesn't take much more time, especially if you already have your onion, celery, and carrots prepped. I think the extra flavor that the mirepoix provides is worth it.

Snacks

Most of my snacks are small, flavor-packed bites that combine salty and sweet flavors. I have found that the more I can activate my palate with different types of flavor, the more satisfied I feel with a food.

Peanut Butter and Raisins

Makes: 1 serving

A little bit of peanut butter goes a long way, but be careful with the amount of peanut butter because it's easy to turn 1 tablespoon into more, and then it becomes a meal instead of a snack.

   1 tablespoon peanut butter
   1 ounce raisins

Sprinkle raisins onto peanut butter and eat. Even though it's just one tablespoon of peanut butter, the full-fat flavor is extremely satisfying to the taste buds. This is my favorite snack to eat with celery, carrot, and broccoli sticks.

Prunes with Honey, Almonds, and Coconut

Makes: 1 serving

I recommend buying the unsulphured prunes because they're not as moist, which makes it a bit more difficult to overeat them. Prunes are roughly 20 calories each, and if you add a nut and some honey, the count goes up by about 12 calories for each treat.

   2–4 prunes
   1 teaspoon honey, for drizzle
   2–4 almonds, or 1 tablespoon unsweetened coconut
   Kosher salt, to sprinkle

To make this sweet treat, drizzle a bit of honey over the prunes, stick an almond on top of each one, or sprinkle unsweetened coconut on top of the honey. A pinch of kosher salt finishes it off nicely.

Maple Cinnamon Parfait

Makes: 1 serving

It always surprises me that 6 ounces of plain yogurt has so few calories, only about 90–120. You can add a handful of raisins or nuts (watch the calories) to this if you'd like a bit of added texture.

    4 ounces plain yogurt
    4 ounces cottage cheese
    1 tablespoon sweetener (maple syrup, brown sugar, or sugar)
    Dash of vanilla extract (optional)
    Cinnamon, to taste

Combine first four ingredients in a bowl and mix well. Top with cinnamon.

Fruit Smarts

To me, apples are the most satisfying fruit; they're delicious and filling thanks to the fibrous skin and dense texture. When choosing fruit for a snack, I like to get the biggest bang for my calorie buck. Oranges are just too high in calories and not enough bulk. Pears are a good choice, but like most fruit, best only when in season. Stone fruits like peaches and nectarines in the summer are always delicious, but if you can't stop at one, then it's best to keep walking. Strawberries and blueberries are great choices, but just be sure to measure them beforehand. Cherries and grapes are the two I know I need to watch, which is why I buy them only in the quantity I want to eat. If you buy a pound, you'll most likely eat a pound, which is 400 calories.

Salad on a Stick

Making Salad on a Stick is a great way to hone your knife skills. Once cleaned and prepped, fresh veggies from the market will last over a week in the fridge. Keep them in a plastic bag with a slightly damp paper towel inside, which will provide just enough moisture to keep them crisp. Once you have your knife and cutting board out, pre-cut all the veggies you have time and energy for. There's nothing nicer than reaching into your fridge on your way out the door and having fresh foods at the ready. Remember: if you don't plan to succeed, you plan to fail.

You can make a beautiful spread by trying any and all farmers' market vegetables you may have never had before. Some of my favorite discoveries are: French radishes, yellow and purple carrots, fresh green beans, orange cauliflower florets, thin asparagus stalks, and yellow bell peppers.

Cut all veggies into sticks ½ inch wide and 3-4 inches long. You can eat as much as you like until the dip runs out. A few vegetable options:

- *Celery*
- *Carrots*
- *Red bell pepper*
- *Baby tomatoes*
- *Radishes*
- *English cucumber*
- *Cauliflower*
- *Broccoli*
- *Green beans*
- *Asparagus*

The last four suggestions can be eaten raw or blanched or steamed slightly, making them more tender. To blanch, bring a large pot of water to a boil, submerge one type of vegetable at a time for 2-4 minutes. Rinse immediately under cold water to stop further cooking.

Dip This Way

To make the dips for my Salad on a Stick, I use one whole container of non-fat FAGE Greek yogurt, to which I add 1 tablespoon of a fat, such as olive oil, mayonnaise, or avocado, and tons of flavor using low- or no-calorie flavor additions.

To prepare any of these dips, simply mix the ingredients in the order they're listed, adding the acid (lime or lemon juice) and salt at the end and tasting to adjust the flavor the way you like it. Each of these dips has about 200 calories and can be enjoyed as one serving or split into two.

Salsa Dip

6–7 ounces plain yogurt

1 tablespoon olive oil or mayonnaise

¾ cup Fresh Salsa (see page 200)

1 garlic clove, pressed

1 lime, juiced, to taste

Salt

Caesar Dip

6 ounces plain yogurt

1 tablespoon mayonnaise

2–4 teaspoons anchovy paste, or minced anchovies

1 garlic clove, pressed

1–2 tablespoons Parmesan cheese

1 lemon, juiced

Basil Tomato Dip

6 ounces plain yogurt

1 tablespoon olive oil, or mayonnaise

1 handful basil, minced

2–3 sundried tomatoes, minced (if packed in oil, reduce olive oil)

1 garlic clove, pressed

Salt

Avocado Lime Dip

6 ounces plain yogurt

1 garlic clove, pressed

1 jalapeño, minced

½ small avocado, mashed

1 lime, juiced, to taste

Goat Cheese and Chive Dip

6 ounces plain yogurt

1 ounce soft goat cheese

1 tablespoon chopped fresh chives

1 lemon, juiced

Salt

Caramelized Onion Dip

6 ounces plain yogurt

½ cup caramelized onions (see page 201; omit red pepper flakes)

½ ounce feta cheese

A splash of red wine vinegar

Salt

Make Them Your Own

Reuse the recipes I've provided for you as often as you can—the more often you make a recipe, the more inclined you are to memorize it quickly. Of course, this is easiest when you pick two or three to really master first. The goal for you should be to eventually cook without a recipe, as this will save you tons of time prepping and cooking. With practice, you will develop the confidence to make the recipe your own by making changes that reflect your personal tastes. Aim to become fast and efficient at feeding yourself—this will not only ensure long-term weight loss, but it will also give you the gift of a lifetime of health.

PART FOUR

You Won the Lottery

13

The First Day of the Rest of Your Life

I always knew I was special. Before you think I'm being arrogant, I want to say this: I think everyone is special, and I think each and every one of you knows it. Somehow we lose sight of this knowledge—maybe it starts early in our childhood with our parents or teachers reminding us of what we don't know or what we can't do, or maybe it doesn't happen until later in life.

Either way, this sense of specialness gets buried within and it begins to feel more natural to believe the doubts and insecurities you have floating around in your head. But guess what? You don't have to believe those destructive thoughts anymore—you are amazing and you know it. With *The Swing!*, you've harnessed the power to change and your greatness has burst onto the scene with all its incredible energy, strength, and confidence—there's no looking back.

After my transformation, the feeling of good fortune grew even stronger. I felt so lucky that I used to think I was going to win the lottery—I used to buy tickets literally convinced that I was going to win. One day, I realized it wasn't the lottery that I was going to win, but something profoundly awesome was definitely going to happen to me. I felt so strongly about this, but I never concerned myself with the details of how or what exactly was going to happen to me, or for me—I just knew.

On one of my walks, I was thinking about this feeling, and it struck me that I had already won—something profound had happened to me—I went through an extraordinary life transformation. I had transformed myself in a way few ever do, at an age when many people have surrendered the hope of ever truly changing their lives. I was a woman in my forties, I felt more alive than ever before, I was more hopeful about my future than I had ever been, I was looking better and feeling more confident than I ever had . . . this was better than the lottery—in fact, it's something that no amount of money can buy.

These days, I think of it more as having discovered a pot of gold because I can look back and see the path I traveled to get here. When I look back, I see the smaller rewards and incentives that kept me going—the little totes of gold—that led up to an endless fortune. I used to think this was a secret, hidden path that only exclusive members knew about, but it's not, and it's a path you're now on, too. You are on this path because you made the choice to honor the gift of your physical body and to treat it with the type of love and attention it deserves—to *stay* on the path, you simply have to continue making the same choices to eat real foods and swing a kettlebell; that's certainly what's kept me here.

Life Without Walls

I never identified with the fat girl I saw in the mirror, and I wondered my whole life why God had made this mistake of putting me in the wrong body. When I used to see my fat reflection, I often found myself doing a double take in disbelief. Being a fat child was like waking up Christmas morning only to discover that Santa had forgotten you, except it happened every morning.

I'm often puzzled when others have the opposite experience—they see a fat person where there isn't one anymore. There are a lot of people who choose to identify with being fat when they are no longer so. Maybe it's their insecurity or a feeling of being undeserving, or maybe they are looking for sympathy or commiseration. Either way, staying married to your overweight identity when you've already separated is just a way of staying stuck—once you've emerged from outside of the shell, don't let the thoughts and trappings of your "before" body keep you mentally stuck. You are free.

If you struggle with breaking free from negative thought patterns, you are not alone—they can be more stubborn than unwanted pounds, but they can be lost just the same, too. Even years after I completely transformed my body, I still fought the labels I had placed on myself in my head; labels like "compulsive eater" or "binge eater" stuck around for much longer than I'd like to admit. The key to overcoming any self-defeating terms or phrases like these that you may have for yourself is consistency—you must consistently and repeatedly deny them anytime they enter your thoughts. When I stopped listening to those labels, they stopped showing up in my actions for good. Instead of thinking it was natural to believe the worst about myself, I began to believe the best about myself, and that's when my thoughts were finally as healthy and fit as my body.

To Cheat or Not to Cheat

Because weight loss comes from creating a calorie deficit, you may be wondering if you can let calorie monitoring and the high-calorie day go once you reach your goal. I don't like to think of myself as forever needing to monitor what I eat, but I do like the idea of keeping data that can give me explanations for changes in my body. I don't need data to tell me when I've gained a little weight, though—I can tell based on how my clothes fit me. And I don't really need data to tell me why my clothes feel tighter—I know it's because I'm eating too many calories, whether I like it or not. Over the years, I have discovered that drifting too far from the principles that changed my life can lead to trouble, or at the very least lead me in the opposite direction of where I know I feel best. Let me tell you a little precautionary tale.

I maintained my lowest average body weight for about three years, and then over the course of a year, I gained back 20 pounds. I lived with the extra weight and felt only mildly upset about it, still never missing a workout or yoga practice. But finally, I reached a point where I had to get a better grasp on what was happening to my body, so I went back to the facts, to the science.

Through my detective work, I discovered that I had started to eat willy-nilly—that is, without a plan. I was still eating my own homemade, high-quality, nutritious foods, but I was eating too much and giving myself too many choices. As soon as I went back to what I already knew, which was to eat the same basic foods in the same basic portions most days of the week, this automatically brought me back to my general calorie range, and 10 pounds dropped off just like that. What about the other 10 pounds?

A little more digging into my eating habits, including looking back at old food journals, helped me realize that I had gotten away from cycling my calories, or including a high-calorie day. I went back to the weekly high-calorie day, and another 3 pounds fell off.

The other 7? I've decided they can come and go, which is something I never thought I would say. I can say this now because I'm within striking range of my lowest average body weight, and because six years of consistent training has built some substantial "muscle density" on my body—that means that even though I may technically weigh more, I'm leaner and stronger than I've ever been. I've grown personally to the point where I know I make the decision of my body weight, and no one else decides that for me. I'm no longer in the dark—I know I have the knowledge, skills, and power to create the body I want, whenever I want, and I have. It's a completely liberating experience.

A lot of people will refer to where you are now as the maintenance phase, but maintenance sounds so clinical and dull to me—you've worked your butt off and gotten to that pot of gold, and now you're just maintaining? You have just started to truly live! You are in the fabulous forever phase—this is permanent. To make sure you stay in this place, rely on your knowledge, and keep your awareness intact—don't drift too high up into the clouds to the point where you forget to apply the rules. Don't think of them as chains but as lifelong partners in extending your prime.

Reflections on Your Former Self

Not too long ago, I found an old pair of jeans that I wore when I weighed 250 pounds. I couldn't believe my body used to be big enough to fit into them, but I didn't look at them and feel shame or embarrassment. When I saw those jeans or I see pictures of myself from so many of those years, I think about how grateful I am for having lost the weight because it allowed me to discover my true self. I am finally, and will forever be, the new and improved version of the best me.

The best part of my whole transformation is that everyone who knew me while I was fat doesn't remember me that way—not even I do. Although some friends who haven't seen me in awhile aren't used to recognizing me the way I am now, it's not because I'm no longer fat, it's because of my energy. Everything I present to the world is different, not just my physical appearance. I'm so happy, confident, and filled with life—that's why they don't recognize me. How cool is that?

As you process and engage in life from a new perspective, honor and appreciate yourself for the progress you've made, for the progress you make every day. Never look back with regret or self-loathing; consider instead that every step you've taken has gotten you to where you are today. You can't pick and choose which parts of yourself or your life to neglect or deny because they all have played a role in creating the incredible you of today.

Perfectly Imperfect

So how do you avoid falling into old patterns? By establishing or creating new, more exciting, and more rewarding patterns. You know, there was a time shortly after I started my diet that I had the thought of never, ever being able to go back to the way I used to eat. I thought about never again eating my everyday lunch of three cheeseburgers and six chocolate chip cookies, and I felt sad for a few moments. I felt like I had just been sentenced to a lifetime of no fun in punishment for my decades of bad behavior.

The sadness passed once I realized how ridiculous it was to mourn the passing of an extremely destructive habit. It dawned on me that it was a lot like feeling sad about the end of an abusive or bad relationship. It's true you might feel sad at first, but then once you've met the person of your dreams, you forget all about the loser you wasted so much of your life with. And if every once in awhile, the jerk gives you a call—hang up! You already know where it's going to lead, and it's nowhere good.

Now that you have the body of your dreams, you'll find yourself not even entertaining the idea of going back to that destructive and neglectful life you used to lead. You have a new love, and it's yourself and your new lifestyle.

Staying in the Zone

Your transformation can be radical and quick, and with it will come the discovery of a whole new physical world. Deciding to try yoga, or training for a walking, biking, or running fundraiser, or even simply wearing sleeveless shirts and trendy workout clothes, aren't just experiences available to other people—it's your turn to have those choices in your life. The more you step into this world of health and fitness and explore it, the more certain you are to stick to your healthy habits.

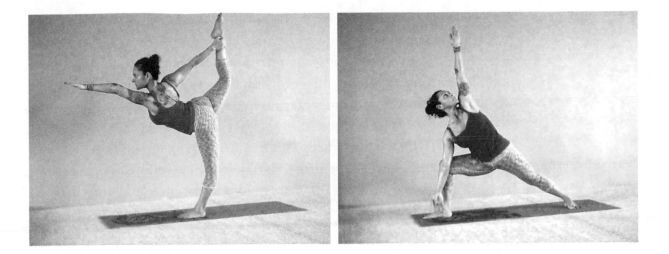

This doesn't mean you have to start running half marathons or swimming through the ocean, but you could if you wanted to. I'm now not only a kettlebell athlete but a yogini too. The question is: who do you want to be?

I like to say that I only took up yoga because I couldn't train with the kettlebell every day, but that's really only part of it. The best part of having a regular yoga practice is being able to say, "I have a regular yoga practice!" I never thought I would have a body that could do yoga regularly and do it well. The day I walked into my first yoga class, I felt no intimidation and I discovered another way to express my newfound confidence. I have the confidence now to take on anything my heart or body desires.

This kind of confidence makes you better at everything you do, whether you have a professional career, are at home raising a family and managing a household, or you're doing all of the above. Before I lost over 100 pounds, my kids couldn't care less about how I looked—they just wanted a ride to school. After I lost the weight and got in shape, they always pointed me out to their friends saying, "That's *my* mom!" Look around you—at your co-workers, at other parents, at people in the grocery store—wherever you are in the outside world, look around and take notice of how many people you see who are of normal weight—and beyond that, who truly look healthy and fit. There aren't that many, which is a shame, but I know you can become one of them. Once you join the club, it will become even more obvious. Keeping your membership is up to you, but you will discover it comes with some incredible, endless rewards.

The rewards are what will keep you inspired, and you will find inspiration comes in many forms. It may come in the form of compliments. It may come in the form of performance, whether it's feeling good about doing something new or getting better at something. It may come in the form of a new pair of jeans. Or it may come in the form of a clean bill of health from your doctor. There is no end to the possibilities.

The greatness doesn't stop there because from inspiration comes motivation, and motivation is contagious. When you travel the path and you reach the pot of gold, you'll see what I mean—it's not something you want to keep to yourself. You will want to shout it out and wave your friends over. You are now the inspiration to others.

Acknowledgments

First and foremost, thanks to Timothy Ferriss for being the generous person that you are, for leading the way and being the inspiration for so many, including me. I'm incredibly grateful for having the chance to work with you. Many, many thanks and much appreciation.

To Pavel Tsatsoline, Chief Instructor RKC, the man responsible for the popularity of kettlebells in this country today: I will always be grateful that you thought to share my story with Tim, proving that a former fat girl can turn into a real deal kettlebell athlete. Thank you for developing your RKC system; it helped me change my life in a way I never thought possible.

Thank you to Steve Hanselman, my agent (I like saying that!), and Julia Serebrinsky, for your unbounded confidence in me, and for taking a risk on an unknown—you brought the dream of this book to life. Without your professional guidance I would not have been able to share this miracle with so many, and so quickly.

To Gretchen Lees, quite possibly the smartest woman I know. Through your tireless work and commitment, you brought greater clarity to my voice without ever compromising truth. You are an amazing writer and truly a professional. You have come to know me better than anyone except my husband Mark and you still like me (I think!). Now, if I could only get you to swing a kettlebell.

To Nancy Hancock, my editor at HarperOne, for agreeing to that first meeting when she asked me why I wanted to write this book. "Because I want this for everyone!" I answered, holding back tears. "This" of course is the greatest feeling of all—to come alive again, and in your best possible body. Thank you, Nancy, for taking the vision of this book and helping craft it into a powerful and polished piece of work.

To DragonDoor and John DuCane for first publishing my story about weight loss and kettlebells. Thanks to you and Pavel for helping to bring the kettlebell to the forefront with the RKC system, and for educating so many on the skill of strength.

All of my blog followers, whose support through kind words and comments you have given me all these years—thank you for inspiring me!

Thank you to all of my students, whom I consider my training partners, for believing like I do that confidence and strength know no age, gender, or weight limits.

To my cooking teachers, who accepted my frantic emergency phone calls in the middle of recipes gone wrong. To Ruth, for always reminding me that, "it's just cooking"—a phrase I still live by in my kitchen.

To my mother, for being the best mom she could be.

And again, I want to acknowledge my husband Mark, to whom this book is dedicated. He's the only man who has ever mattered in my life and I will forever be *his* biggest fan.

Finally, to all the chubby little girls and boys who have had to sit on the sidelines knowing they are capable of so much more, and to everyone who has ever felt underestimated: you know you have greatness within you—bring it to life and stop waiting for another day—today is the day!

Appendix A

The Swing!	DAILY EATING JOURNAL	
DATE:		

Meal 1:	Veggies:	Time:
	Protein:	
	Fat:	
	Carbs:	
Meal 2:	Veggies:	Time:
	Protein:	
	Fat:	
	Carbs:	
Meal 3:	Veggies:	Time:
	Protein:	
	Fat:	
	Carbs:	
Snacks:		Time:

WORKOUT:
Activity:

NOTES:

Appendix B

Use these journals for Workouts #1–5 and #14–15. For Workouts #6–13, follow instructions directly from pages 139 to 143 in Chapter 9.

The Swing!	OTM WORKOUT #1		
Swings	**Sets**	**Sets Completed**	**Work/Rest**
10 2- hd sw	5		
8–10 2-hd sw	5		
5–10 2-hd sw	5		
Total Workout Time: 15 minutes			
Notes:			

The Swing!	OTM WORKOUT #2		
Swings	**Sets**	**Sets Completed**	**Work/Rest**
10 2-hd sw	5		
_____ 2-hd sw	1		
_____ 2-hd sw	1		
_____ 2-hd sw	1		
_____ 2-hd sw	1		
_____ 2-hd sw	1		
_____ 2-hd sw	5		

Total Workout Time: 15 minutes

Notes:

The Swing!	OTM WORKOUT #3		
Swings	**Sets**	**Sets Completed**	**Work/Rest**
10 2-hd sw	5		
_____ 2-hd sw	1		
_____ 2-hd sw	1		
_____ 2-hd sw	1		
_____ 2-hd sw	1		
_____ 2-hd sw	1		
_____ 2-hd sw	1		
_____ 2-hd sw	1		
_____ 2-hd sw	1		
_____ 2-hd sw	1		
_____ 2-hd sw	1		
_____ 2-hd sw	5		

Total Workout Time: 20 minutes

Notes:

The Swing!	OTM WORKOUT #4		
Swings	**Sets**	**Sets Completed**	**Work/Rest**
12 2-hd sw	1		
____ 2-hd sw	1		
____ 2-hd sw	1		
____ 2-hd sw	1		
____ 2-hd sw	1		
____ 2-hd sw	1		
____ 2-hd sw	1		
____ 2-hd sw	1		
____ 2-hd sw	1		
____ 2-hd sw	1		
20 2-hd sw	10–15		

Total Workout Time: 20–25 minutes

Notes:

The Swing!	OTM WORKOUT #5		
Swings	**Sets**	**Sets Completed**	**Work/Rest**
12 2-hd sw	1		
____ 2-hd sw	1		
____ 2-hd sw	1		
____ 2-hd sw	1		
____ 2-hd sw	1		
20 2-hd sw	10–20		
____ 2-hd sw	10		

Total Workout Time: 25–30 minutes

Notes:

The Swing!	WORKOUT #14		
Swings	**Sets**	**Rest**	**Actual Rest**
10 2-hd sw	1	15 seconds	
10 R/10 L	1	30 seconds	
5 R/5 L	3	45 seconds	
40 2-hd sw	1	1 minute	
50 TR	1	1.25 minutes	
60 SW/TR	1	1.5 minutes	
5 R/5 L	7	1.75 minutes	
10 R/10 L	4	2 minutes	
5 R/5 L	6	1.5 minutes	
40 SW/TR	1	1 minute	
20 TR	1	30 seconds	
10 2-hd sw	1	DONE!	

Total Workout Time: 18–24 minutes

Notes:

The Swing! WORKOUT #15

Swings	Sets	Rest	Actual Rest
10 2-hd sw	1	15 seconds	
20 2-hd sw	1	30 seconds	
30 2-hd sw	1	45 seconds	
40 2-hd sw	1	1 minute	
50 TR	1	1.25 minutes	
60 SW/TR	1	1.5 minutes	
5 R/5 L × 2	7	1.75 minutes	
10 R/10 L	8	2 minutes	
5 R/5 L	8	2 minutes	
80 SW/TR	1	2 minutes	
80 TR	1	2 minutes	
40 2-hd sw	1	DONE!	

Total Workout Time: 21–28 minutes

Notes:

About the Author

At the age of forty-one, after having been overweight her entire life, Tracy Reifkind lost 120 pounds and discovered a path to lasting transformation using kettlebells. She is now a sought-after personal trainer and motivation and nutrition coach who was featured in Tim Ferriss's *The 4-Hour Body.* In 2006, she became a certified Russian kettlebell instructor. Since then, she has developed a unique training program that works for anyone, at any fitness level, featured in her DVD "Programming the Kettlebell Swing." Reifkind lives in California with her husband, Mark. They have two grown sons.

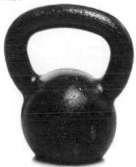